Problem-Oriented Pediatric Diagnosis

Problem-Oriented Pediatric Diagnosis

Roger M. Barkin, M.D., M.P.H.

Chairman, Department of Pediatrics, Rose Medical Center; Associate Professor of Pediatrics and Surgery, University of Colorado Health Sciences Center

Little, Brown and Company
Boston/Toronto/London

First Edition

Library of Congress Catalog
Card No. 90-60953
ISBN 0-316-08102-7

Printed in the United States of America
SEM

Third Printing

Contents

Preface

One of the most exciting components of clinical pediatrics is the many differential considerations in approaching a clinical problem with which a patient presents. Each patient presents with a unique combination of complaints, concerns, anxieties, and past history that allow the clinician to begin to clarify possible contributing medical conditions. In the pediatric patient, this is often more difficult because the parents and other care providers are the historians and observers rather than the patient. The child is often frightened, and the history rarely provides specific data on which to focus a diagnostic and therapeutic plan. Children consistently present in a nonspecific fashion and make the differential diagnosis broader and more difficult, requiring a high level of clinical acumen and understanding.

Problem-Oriented Pediatric Diagnosis focuses on *problems* rather than diagnostic entities and systems, thereby facilitating the movement from presenting signs and symptoms, to diagnosis, and ultimately to treatment. This closely parallels the analytical process of pediatrics. For clinicians in every stage of training and practice, this is a truly challenging, yet problematic, area and requires specific attention. Specific clinical entities can be easily accessed by using the extensive index.

First, it is essential to define the nature of the problem and potential etiologic considerations. A systematic approach must be developed, including a complete and relevant history. Complaints should be defined with respect to the onset, progression, nature, associated signs and symptoms, activities or treatments that worsen or ameliorate the problem, and recurrences. The physical should be complete and focus on areas of specific complaint as well as components that may be useful in differential considerations. Common and important conditions are outlined in the etiologic consideration tables.

Subsequently, an appropriate diagnostic approach must be outlined. Laboratory and radiologic evaluation may be confirmatory. Often a therapeutic trial may be useful in excluding certain considerations.

We make no attempt to be comprehensive with respect to the pathophysiology of the problems covered but present material that is useful to you, the clinician, in approaching specific clinical presentations. In understanding the ill child, it is also essential to have an understanding of normal growth and development, which is the focus of the initial chapter.

Management is not discussed because of the diagnostic focus of this book and the ready availability of such strategies in other references. Appendixes are included to assist in defining normals and additionally provide general information about managing common ailments.

Medical and traumatic illnesses may progress rapidly in the pediatric patient, but the vast majority are treatable and the child is generally expected to recover without sequelae and with a full life ahead. This provides the ultimate challenge and the true opportunity in caring for the pediatric patient.

We hope that you find this book useful in approaching clinical problems and understanding the breadth and depth of pediatric diagnostic considerations. Whether in training or in practice, this book should facilitate the assessment of complex patients, as well as those with more routine presentations. Use it to expand your horizons and make medicine more fun.

R.M.B.

Acknowledgments

One's clinical acumen and judgment is largely the synthesis of the many physicians, nurses, children, and parents who have provided two decades of learning and clinical experience.

I am grateful to the Rose Children's Center at Rose Medical Center, Denver, and the Departments of Pediatrics and Surgery at the University of Colorado Health Sciences Center for their ongoing support during the development of this book.

Susan Pioli, Kristin Odmark, Priscilla Hurdle, Nan Nagy, and Kathi Thompson's unending support and frequent reminders made this book move smoothly through its many phases to completion.

I The Pediatric Patient

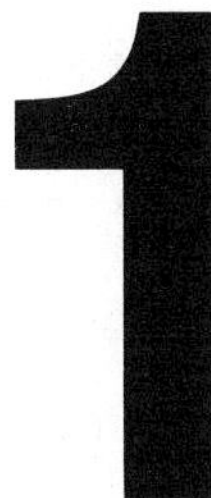

Approaching the Healthy Child

Routine visits are an integral part of providing ongoing information about child care and parenting. These visits are important to help ensure that a child is growing and developing normally and is being protected from a variety of infections. These are times of friendly and positive interaction, allowing the health care provider to make observations, answer questions, and get additional perspective on a child's normal growth and development while at the same time reassuring parents and reducing anxiety. Approach the child by observing, playing, and cajoling before undertaking the more unpleasant parts of the exam such as examining the ears and throat.

At each visit, children are weighed and measured: weight, height, and frontal-occipital circumference (FOC). Their development is assessed, special issues and concerns are discussed, and a physical examination is performed. Immunizations are administered according to a specific schedule. The child's growth parameters are plotted to determine that his or her growth pattern is appropriate and following a specific and normal curve (Appendix B). Development will also be assessed through screening tests and careful examinations.

The *two week visit* provides an opportunity to ensure that the new baby, parents, and other siblings are adjusting well. The child will have normally regained birthweight. It is an excellent time to ask questions about feeding, bowel movements, urination, sleeping, sibling rivalry, and safety precautions. Discuss frustrations and fatigue also. A second phenylketonuria (PKU) test is performed.

At *2*, *4*, and *6 months* of age, the baby is again weighed. Direct particular attention toward the adjustment of the family, any problems or conflicts, accident prevention, and development. Diphtheria-tetanus-pertussis (DTP) and polio vaccines are administered (Table 1-1).

No immunizations are given at *9 months* of age, but growth and development are assessed. Discuss parenting concerns.

At *1 year*, accident prevention and growth and development are assessed. Specific areas of frustration or concern are the focus.

The next immunization is scheduled at *15–18 months* of age. Measles-mumps-rubella (MMR) vaccine as well as DTP and polio are recommended. Haemophilus influenzae (HIB) conjugate vaccine is also given (Table 1-1). Discuss accident and poison prevention, behavior, weaning, discipline, toilet training, and other potential frustrations.

At *2 years*, discuss behavior and safety while assessing growth and development.

Table 1-1. Recommended Immunization Schedule

Age	Immunization
2 months	DTP, polio
4 months	DTP, polio
6 months	DTP
15–18 months	DTP, polio, MMR, HIB
4–5 years	DTP, polio

From *3 to 5 years* of age children are seen annually to reassess growth and development and deal with questions about discipline and behavior. Safety issues are of particular concern, including street, bicycle, and water safety. Additional DTP and polio are administered at 5 years of age and dental visits are initiated (Table 1-1).

Behavior as a Developmental Process

Each encounter is an opportunity to observe the child and speak with parents as well as to assess the child's growth and development and provide counsel and assistance. It is essential to understand behavior and its developmental aspects.

Understanding basic principles is necessary for a developmental approach to behavior modification. Occasionally it is necessary to redirect children's activity and redefine appropriate limits; *consistency* must be the basis for all such efforts. Expectations and limits should be appropriate for the child's development. Two-year-olds should not be asked to sit still at a meeting for two hours, entertain themselves while their parents get the housework done, or go out to a fancy restaurant and be "angels."

Parents should listen to, respect, and give children room for exploration. But parents must also make sure their children know their limits and they must be decisive when setting boundaries. Within this framework, children need reassurance and praise to allow them to develop independence while still understanding that there are boundaries that cannot be broken.

Consistent boundaries allow children to be secure enough to wander and push their curiosity while accepting the authority, love, and security provided by their parents. Without clear limits, children will not know their boundaries, and they often become insecure about their relationships with adults and their environment. Although these limits are good for children, parents should not expect thank-yous for setting early bedtimes.

Limits must be set; it is essential to be consistent while providing a positive, loving and caring environment. Defining clear and concise boundaries will help to establish appropriate behavior, and children will feel safer.

Consistency and support are particularly important in helping children deal with the fear of the unknown. The vivid imagination of children may lead to distortion of reality and unfounded fears, and consistent limits can help children to structure and reformulate.

It is not always easy to be consistent; children will constantly test limits and attempt to circumvent the rules. Persistence is required – even though there may be doubts! A sense of humor and perspective is essential. The hard times are always followed by good ones; the converse is true as well.

Children will also reflect the values and support system with which they are surrounded. A secure environment must be provided; nevertheless there will be times of variable stress. At even the youngest age, children reflect household tension and will manifest their sense of discomfort and insecurity by changing behavior, often becoming more demanding.

Even children under a year of age understand the word "No," particularly when it is said in a firm voice. They respond to the communication, even if they do not understand the term; if the child does not respond immediately, isolating him or her will provide added emphasis. Older children clearly understand the term. They tend to want to test limits and will often say "No," automatically, regardless of the nature of the request. Children at this stage say "No" to even the most tempting offers of ice cream or candy, just as a "matter of principle."

After 18 months of age, children often need periods to cool down and think about their actions. This is an excellent place to adopt a *quiet time* to change behavior. This works immeasurably better than spanking or threatening because those approaches are short lived, and to some extent they demonstrate the child's control. Parents should be teachers, not police officers.

Quiet times allow children to have time alone after some unacceptable behavior, such as disobeying, throwing a tantrum, biting, yelling, or any of a host of other infractions. Parents should use identical responses for similar behaviors and define which behaviors warrant a quiet time. Parents must explain to their children in a calm voice what they have done to warrant a quiet time. Quiet time should take place in a predetermined, nonstimulating site. A timer is often helpful. If the child leaves the chair, the timer is reset. Once the quiet time is over and the child is ready to get up, forget the episode and begin again on a positive note. Expectations must be age-appropriate, and allowances must be made for changes and variants that are really normal behavior. If behavioral problems escalate or parents or children are getting frustrated, counseling and support may be necessary.

The Developing Child

Watch children grow throughout the early years; it is perhaps the most amazing and exciting part of raising children. Babies are unique and during the first two years of life gain skills with a rapidity that is astounding. Each day new things are learned, new behaviors are evident, and new sounds and responses are present. *Part of the excitement is that all children develop on somewhat different time tables. Although the pattern and general framework are consistent, the variability makes it fun and full of surprises.*

Normal development provides insights into behavior. Children adopt behaviors that may occasionally be frustrating but are usually a part of *normal* development. Independence, separation anxiety, and jealousy are recurrent themes that form the basis for many developmental changes that have an impact on behavior. *Most behaviors that are considered problematic are actually exaggerations of normal development and may be a reflection of the variability that exists among children in acquiring new skills.* It is essential to recognize this in encouraging children to take age-appropriate risks and challenges that allow them to explore and experiment. Supporting and encouraging growth and the expansion of horizons leads to self-confidence.

Newborn

Babies arrive with anticipation and fanfare. Increasingly, new babies can interact with their environment. Although babies have little control of muscles and can barely (if at all) hold their heads up, they have an amazing ability to look at their environment and respond to people, sounds, colors, and shapes. Babies follow to the midline and enjoy looking at faces and are occasionally interactive with bright, shiny, moving objects. They should be talked to, played with, and entertained.

The early weeks are ones of bonding with mother and father and siblings. There are intense time demands: feedings to give, diapers to change, and laundry to do. These fill the time between enjoying the baby and ensuring that other children are included and that spouses are not forgotten. Everyone must be part of the excitement and get pleasure from the new arrival while some semblance of family functioning is maintained. Schedules and demands from neighbors, friends, in-laws, and work can be a phenomenal drain and must be kept in perspective.

Six Weeks

Children by 6 weeks are increasingly able to do things and respond in a more positive and animated way to sounds, faces, actions, and so on. Even as newborns, babies are taking it all in; they are just not responding. By 6 weeks some children are making some sounds and smile in response to faces. They now follow past the midline.

Interactive playing is essential. Babies follow brightly colored objects better and even make early attempts at grabbing things. However, they will not hold them or play with them in a consistent manner.

Babies sleep continuously but now there is more responsiveness, and more noises are made; part of this becomes a response to the actions of others. They feed with somewhat more purpose and are less passive in terms of position and demands.

Four Months

By this time, the 4-month-old is sociable and responds with an exciting array of faces, sounds, and motions to every word. The baby makes sounds constantly, like squeals, coos, and babbles either because he or she gets pleasure from the noise or to get a response from someone. Now babies will respond to most people who are willing to play, crawl, squeal, or make funny faces. Smiling becomes more common.

Muscle control improves and there is more physical interaction with the environment. Children look at their hands and grab for things and are able to grasp an object with a wide swing of the arms and hands. They slowly develop an ability for self-support while in someone's arms or in an infant seat. One of the most exciting events is when a child finally turns over. Often the baby will not understand what has just happened and begin to cry after this tremendous feat. There is also some evidence that babies enjoy being held in a standing position, although obviously they cannot do this without assistance. All of this increased control allows children to entertain themselves and keep track of what is going on in a more active fashion. Interest is still primarily in people.

Six Months

Six-month-olds are constantly exploring. Eyes, fingers, hands, and mouth become essential parts of this process. Everything is new and needs to be felt, looked at, tasted, and chewed. Things can now be grabbed with more skill and even transferred from one hand to another. Cubes are common playtoys. All of a sudden children become social beings, making sounds for themselves or anyone who will respond. Sitting becomes an important landmark at this age and it may happen all of a sudden. Children are in constant motion, but crawling is limited by the inability to keep the stomach off the floor.

Nine Months

Increasingly, interaction with the world becomes more sophisticated. Body movements become more purposeful, usually in moving toward something that appears attractive. Standing is accomplished while they hold on to something. Babies reach out to learn about things, places, and people. Picking up objects and touching everything becomes commonplace. The index finger and thumb can now work together in an efficient pincer action, and the baby's world is thereby expanded immeasurably.

For baby, being included in everything is essential; games such as peek-a-boo are fun. At least the tone of "No" is understood. Sounds are made in a meaningful fashion and "Dada" and "Mama," as well as imitation sounds, become incorporated into the language pattern. Children will listen to readings of books with pictures for longer periods of time. Stranger anxiety becomes a dominant force. Parents are clearly preferred to everyone else and children who a month earlier loved anyone holding them and paying attention now cry whenever someone else picks them up. There is tremendous variability in this stage and it will pass. It is part of the development toward being a healthy, independent person.

Sitting is now perfected; children also scoot or crawl, permitting mobility that is astounding. Many children never crawl much if they can scoot efficiently. Remember that the object is to get from one place to another, not necessarily acquire skills that are not needed. Children enjoy standing up while holding on to some object.

Twelve Months

The first birthday is a landmark, and walking is the big achievement; children may not become efficient walkers for a few more months. The pincer grasp has improved and playing with cubes and other objects is more sophisticated.

Communication skills have escalated and single words, especially "Mama" and "Dada" are clearly understood. Simple directions are understood and limit setting becomes a reality. Children are much more responsive, waving goodbye and wanting to do things by themselves. They now have the ability to ambulate and find things; feeding is often a balance of the child wanting to hold the spoon while combining, smearing, and spilling foods. Dependency is still paramount. Although they like to do things by themselves, separation is still difficult. The security of the favorite blanket is essential and often parents need to stay by the crib for a few minutes until the child has gone to sleep.

Mobility is essential and becomes a part of the child's desire to explore and be independent, but the child still always wants the security of a loved one around. Providing an area that is safe to explore is helpful in assisting in this growth.

Eighteen Months

The 18-month-old is an explorer whose world has expanded over the last few months. Walking has opened a whole new world and when combined with crawling leaves no place safe from the curiosity and initiative of the youngster. There is a tremendous sense of independence and a much greater focus on what he or she really wants. Separation from parents is now more acceptable, but frequent checks for eye contact are reassuring.

Behavior becomes somewhat inconsistent; children may develop fears of certain things, such as baths or loud noises. "No" becomes an important part of an expanded vocabulary, particularly when desires are not met. Often children demonstrate their temper and displeasure with these limits. Diverting attention to more acceptable activities is usually easy at this age. Now is when consistency is important in internalizing appropriate behavior patterns for children.

Vocabulary has increased to several other single words and there is constant babbling. Words are imitated and usually one or more body parts are incorporated into normal play. Playing with friends is now more fun, although it is often done in parallel, with minimal interaction with peers. Often children will get frustrated when they cannot do something; diverting attention may be useful. Children can turn pages by themselves and they like to draw and scribble. They can partially undress themselves at this time.

Two Years

Independence is the hallmark of the 2-year-old who is trying to build new skills and competencies. Two-year-olds want to do everything themselves and get things exactly their way. They want choices, and these should be given when appropriate (i.e., a choice of what clothes to wear but not a choice about when to go to bed or eat). The 2-year-old has emblazoned the word "No" on all communications. Periodically, these intense feelings of independence do give way to a need to be held, praised, and supported; enjoy these moments while they last.

Obviously, children can now move around with tremendous skill, even using tricycles. Balls can be kicked, steps climbed, and objects jumped. Vocabulary gets increasingly sophisticated and sentences can be understood and words combined. Pictures can often be named and body parts identified. Cooperative play and sharing remain limited. Listening to stories is a favorite activity, as is helping with housework.

Three Years

These preschoolers can now pedal the tricycle and go upstairs alternating steps. They enjoy playing with blocks and can even stack them. Balls can usually be thrown overhand a small distance. Copying drawings is tremendous fun. Speech is more understandable and children can describe pictures by combining different objects and describing the action within the story. They enjoy buttoning their clothes and can wash and dry their hands. They can begin to brush their teeth independently (but often forget unless reminded and supervised). Play is more interactive. Masturbation may occur.

Four Years

Hopping is a favorite activity and sense of balance markedly improves. People increasingly become the subject of their drawings and they still love to copy and imitate pictures. Speech is totally understandable and naming opposites is a favorite game. "Why," "how," and "when" are constantly included in all questions and should be recognized as important parts of the learning process.

Children can usually dress themselves with help and many are toilet trained. Separation from parents is easier and play groups work cooperatively.

Five to Eight Years

Balancing is now possible and so is playing with a bounced ball with improved eye-hand coordination and increased speed. Drawings of people are more complicated, including multiple body parts. Exploring is paramount and constant. More control of their environment is expected and greater self-reliance is observed. Increasing group activities, sports, and diversions are requested.

Language is tremendously important and children know body parts; vocabulary is expanded and counting improves.

They can dress themselves.

Watch, enjoy the child. Share in the wonder while guiding the family through the ups and downs, the delights and frustrations. Monitor the child's growth and development and provide protection from infections, accidents, and injury in this process.

Bibliography

American Academy of Pediatrics: *Report of the Committee on Infectious Diseases*, 21st edition. Elk Grove: American Academy of Pediatrics, 1988.

Barkin RM: *The Father's Guide: Raising a Healthy Child*. Golden: Fulcrum, 1988.

Spock B, Rothenberg M: *Dr. Spock's Baby and Child Care*. New York: Pocket Books, 1985.

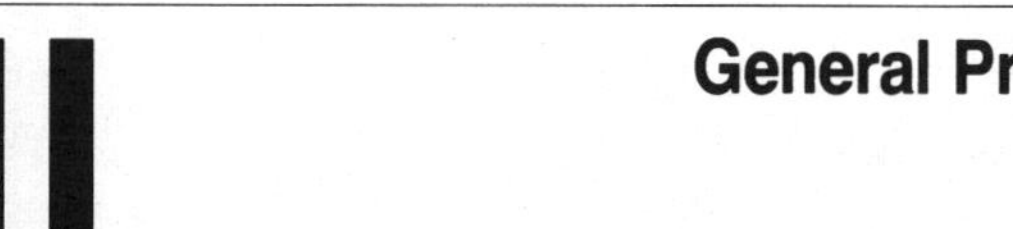

II General Problems

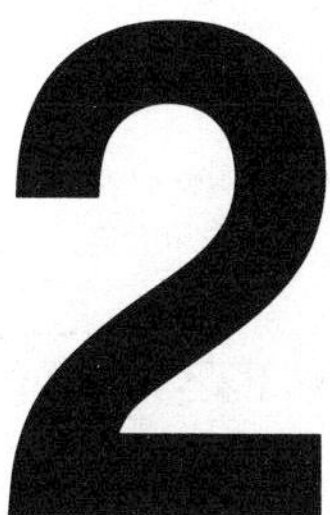

Resuscitating the Child

Cardiopulmonary arrest in children can often be anticipated, thereby preventing progressive deterioration of respiratory, and ultimately circulatory, status. Respiratory illness is usually primary, hypoxia or obstruction eventually leading to cardiac arrest. Awareness and attention to the evidence of respiratory distress can allow early intervention and prevent progression.

Precipitating causes include:

1. Respiratory.
   a. Upper airway obstruction: croup, foreign body, epiglottitis, trauma.
   b. Lower airway disease: pneumonia, asthma, bronchiolitis, foreign body.
2. Infection: sepsis or meningitis.
3. Intoxication: narcotics, sedatives.
4. Cardiac disorder: congenital condition, pericarditis, myocarditis.
5. Shock.
   a. Hypovolemic: gastroenteritis, burns, trauma.
   b. Cardiogenic: congestive heart failure, dysrhythmia.
   c. Distributive: sepsis, anaphylaxis.
6. CNS: meningitis, encephalitis, head trauma, anoxia.
7. Trauma/environment: accident, child abuse, hypothermia, hyperthermia, near-drowning.
8. Metabolic: hypoglycemia, hypocalcemia, hyperkalemia.
9. Near sudden-infant death syndome (SIDS).

Newborns commonly experience catastrophic events due to prematurity, uteroplacental insufficiency, congenital malformation, or sepsis. *Infants* may suffer near-SIDS, child abuse, pulmonary or congenital heart disease, ingestion, and sepsis. *Older children* experience arrests from trauma, intoxication, dysrhythmias, and congenital heart or pulmonary disease.

Basic Life Support

The basic ABCs form the foundation for initial intervention. Stabilizing the *airway*, ensuring adequate *breathing*, and supporting *circulation* are essential.

1. Establish unresponsiveness or respiratory difficulty. Gently shake the child if he or she is unresponsive.
2. Call for help.
3. Position the patient supine on a firm, flat surface such as a board or the floor.
4. Position to open the *airway* using the head tilt-chin lift method, placing head in "sniffing" position.
5. Assess *breathing* by chest and abdominal movement or feeling nasal or oral air movement.
6. If the child is not breathing, initiate mouth to mouth or mouth to nose breathing. Give two slow breaths and if chest moves continue rescue breathing. If there is no air movement, consider whether there is a foreign body obstruction.

   If you suspect an upper airway foreign body and the child is an infant, deliver four back blows and subsequent chest thrust. In a child over 1 year of age, perform Heimlich or abdominal thrust. Repeat until obstruction is relieved.

7. Assess *circulation* by feeling pulse at brachial, femoral, or carotid artery.
8. Begin chest compressions if there is no pulse.
9. Coordinate compressions and breathing using a 5:1 compression to ventilation ratio.
10. Frequently reassess to define response to basic life support.

Advanced Life Support

Following initial basic life support, more sophisticated measures can be introduced to stabilize airway, breathing, and circulation. There are certain considerations that are unique to children.

1. Children primarily have respiratory pathology as the primary condition leading to hypoxia, acidosis, and then circulatory failure. Children may also have primary hypovolemia, which responds to fluids therapy.
2. All fluids, catheters, tubes, drugs, and medications must be age and weight specific. Aggressive monitoring may be required.
3. Fluid resuscitation must also reflect size and weight. Normally, the initial bolus should be 20 ml/kg of normal saline or lactated ringer's over 20–30 minutes, which may be repeated. Intravascular volume is considered to be 80 ml/kg.
4. Children are developing physically and psychologically and the team must be responsive to the needs of the child and family.

Airway patency can be established through a variety of techniques, the options being more limited if there is a question of neck trauma. Adjunctive techniques include one or more of the following:

1. Oxygen administered at 3–6 l/min by mask or cannula.
2. Oropharyngeal airway, which is tolerated well in unconscious patients.
3. Nasopharyngeal airway is tolerated fairly well in conscious patients.
4. Self-inflating bag-valve ventilation, often with oxygen reservoir to enhance oxygen concentration.
5. Endotracheal or nasotracheal intubation provides an efficient, stable airway.

Breathing is demonstrated by chest and abdominal movement or feeling air movement through the nasal or oral areas. Ventilatory support can be effectively provided using a self-inflating bag-valve ventilation system in conjunction with maintenance of the airway.

Circulatory status may be assessed by brachial, femoral, or carotid pulses, blood pressure, heart rate, and capillary refilling (normally < 2 sec). Besides external chest compression, fluid administration may be mandatory and is achieved by intravenous cannulation and rapid administration of fluid (see Chapter 3). The intraosseous (bone marrow) route of infusion is an alternative in life-threatened children under 3 years of age who require fluid administration. Rarely are atropine, epinephrine, lidocaine, or beta-adrenergic agents needed in the initial resuscitation (Table 2-1).

Appropriate monitoring of electrolytes, acidosis, hematocrit, urine output, and vital signs, etc. should be done initially and on an ongoing basis.

Alert: Prevention and early recognition is the key to the management of the seriously ill child. Airway, breathing, and circulation must be stabilized.

Table 2-1. Pediatric Emergency Measures

Drug	Dose
Albuterol (Ventolin, Proventil)	(0.5% soln): 0.01–0.03 ml (0.05–0.15 mg)/kg/dose (max: 0.5 ml/dose) inhalation. May repeat.
Atropine	(0.1, 0.4, 1.0 mg/ml): 0.01–0.03 mg/kg/dose (min: 0.1 mg/dose) (adult: 0.6 – 1.0 mg/dose; max: 2 mg) q 2–5 min prn IV (or ET)
Bicarbonate, sodium	($NaHCO_3$) (44, 50 mEq/50 ml): 1–2 mEq/kg/dose q 10 min prn (per ABG) IV (diluted 1:1 with D5W)
Calcium chloride	(10%: 100 mg/ml–1.36 mEq Ca^{++}/ml): 20–30 mg/kg/dose (max: 500 mg/dose) q 10 min prn IV slowly
Crystalloid	(D5WLR, D5W 0.9% NS, LR, 0.9% NS): 20 ml/kg over 20–30 min IV
Defibrillation	1–2 joules/kg/dose (adult: 200 joules/dose); synchronized: 0.5–1 joules/kg/dose
Dexamethasone (Decadron)	(4, 24 mg/ml): 0.25 mg/kg/dose IV, IM
Dextrose	(D50W: 25 g/50 ml often diluted to D25W): 0.5–1.0 g (2–4 ml D25W)/kg/dose IV
Diazepam (Valium)	(5 mg/ml): 0.2–0.3 mg/kg/dose q 2–5 min prn IV slowly (max total dose: child, 10 mg; adult, 30 mg)
Diazoxide (Hyperstat)	(15 mg/ml): 1–3 mg/kg/dose (max: 150 mg/dose) q 4–24 hr IV rapidly
Digoxin	0.01–0.04 mg/kg total digitalizing dose (TDD) IV reflecting age (adult: 0.5–1.0 mg TDD)
Dopamine	(40, 80, 160 mg/ml): 5–20 μg/kg/min IV drip (6 mg × wt (kg) in 100 ml D5W: 1 ml/hr = 1 μg/kg/min)
Dobutamine (Dobutrex)	(250 mg/vial): 1–15 μg/kg/min IV drip (6 mg × wt (kg) in 100 ml D5W; 1 ml/hr = 1 μg/kg/min)
Epinephrine	*Asystole* (1:10,000): 0.1 ml/kg/dose (max: 5 ml) q 3–5 min prn IV or ET)/; *Asthma* (1:1000):0.01 ml/kg/dose (max: 0.35 ml/dose) q 20 min prn × 3, SQ
Furosemide (Lasix)	(10 mg/ml): 1 mg (max: 6 mg)/kg/dose q 6–12 hr IV
Hydralazine (Apresoline)	(20 mg/ml): 0.1–0.2 mg/kg/dose q 4–6 hr prn IV, IM (adult: 10–20 mg/dose)
Insulin, regular	DKA: 0.1–0.2 units/kg/hr IV drip
Isoproterenol	(200 μg/ml): 0.05–1.5 μg/kg/min IV drip (0.6 mg × wt (kg) in 100 ml D5W; 1 ml/hr = 0.1 μg/kg/min)
Lidocaine	(10, 20 mg/ml): Load: 1 mg/kg/dose q 5–10 min prn IV (or ET) (max total dose: 5 mg/kg); maint: 20–50 μg/kg/min IV drip (adult: 2–4 mg/min)
Lorazepam (Ativan)	(2, 4 mg/ml); 0.05–0.15 mg/kg/dose IV slowly (max: 5 mg/dose)

Table 2-1. Pediatric Emergency Measures (*continued*)

Drug	Dose
Mannitol	(200, 250 mg/ml); 0.25–0.5 g/kg/dose q 3–4 hr prn IV slowly
Methylprednisolone (Solu-Medrol)	(40, 125, 500, 1,000 mg/vial): *Asthma*: 1–2 mg/kg/dose q 6 hr IV.
Morphine	(8, 10, 15 mg/ml): 0.1–0.2 mg/kg/dose (max: 15 mg/dose) q 2–4 hr prn IV, IM
Naloxone (Narcan)	(0.4, 1 mg/ml): 0.1 mg/kg/dose (max: 0.8 mg) IV; if no response in 10 min give 2 mg IV
Nitroprusside (Nipride)	(50 mg/vial): 0.5–10 μg (avg: 3 μg)/kg/min IV drip (50 mg in 100 ml D5W = 500 μg/ml)
Pancuronium (Pavulon)	(1, 2 mg/ml): 0.04–0.1 mg/kg/dose IV; repeat 0.01–0.02 mg/kg/dose q 20–40 min prn IV
Phenobarbital	(65, 130 mg/ml); Load: 15 mg/kg/dose PO, IM, IV (<25–50 mg/min or <1 mg/kg/min) (adult: 100 mg/dose q 20 min prn × 3); maint: 3–5 mg/kg/24 hr PO, IV
Phenytoin (Dilantin)	(50 mg/ml): *Seizure*: Load: 15 mg/kg PO, IV (<40 mg/min or <0.5 mg/kg/min) (Max: 1,250 mg); maint: 5 mg/kg/24 hr PO, IV. *Dysrhythmia*: 5 mg/kg/dose q 5–20 min prn IV
Propranolol (Inderal)	(1 mg/ml): *Dysrhythmia*: 0.01–0.1 mg/kg/dose (max: 1 mg/dose) IV over 10 min. *Tetralogy spell*: 0.1–0.2 mg/kg/dose q 15 min prn IV
Succinylcholine (Anectine)	(20 mg/ml): 1 mg/kg/dose IV; repeat 0.3–0.6 mg/kg/dose q 5–10 min prn IV
Terbutaline (Brethine)	(0.1% soln): 0.01 ml/kg/dose SQ q 20 min × 3 (max: 0.25 ml/dose). Inhalation: 0.03 ml/kg/dose in 2 ml saline (max: 0.5 ml/dose)
Theophylline	(0.85 aminophylline): Load: 5–6 mg/kg IV slowly; maint: 0.6–0.9 mg/kg/hr IV drip

Bibliography

Blumer JL: Pediatric Cardiopulmonary Resuscitation: A Study of Consonant Dissonance. In Barkin RM (ed), *Emergently Ill Child.* Rockville, MD: Aspen Pub, 1987.

Chameides L: *Textbook of Pediatric Advanced Life Support*, Dallas: American Heart Association, 1988.

Eisenberg M, Bergner L, and Hallstrom A: Epidemiology of cardiac arrest and resuscitation in children. Ann Emerg Med 12:672, 1983.

Mayer TA: Emergency pediatric vascular access: old solutions to an old problem. Am J Emerg Med 4:98, 1986.

Spivey W: Intraosseous infusions. J Pediatr 111:639, 1987.

Zaritsky A, Nadkami V, Getsen P, et al.: CPR in children. Ann Emerg Med 16:1107, 1987.

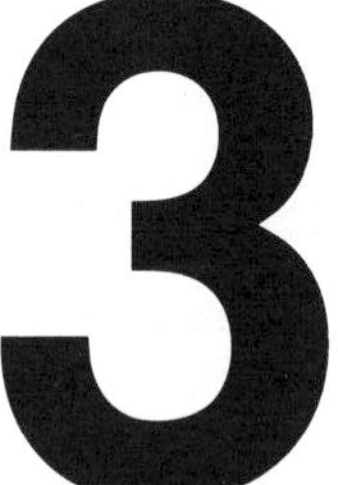

3 Shock

Shock results from acute circulatory failure and cellular dysfunction, and is marked by progressive impairment of blood flow to skin, muscles, kidneys, mesentery, lungs, heart, and brain. When shock occurs, considerations must include fluid deficit, pump failure, resistance changes, and respiratory failure. Respiratory failure may be secondary to cardiovascular dysfunction or may produce circulatory failure with progressive acidosis and hypoxia.

Blood pressure reflects cardiac output and arteriolar resistance. Cardiac output is affected by heart rate and stroke volume, the latter being altered by variations in the preload, afterload, and cardiac contractility. These factors allow the body to compensate for changes in intravascular volume and cardiac function.

Etiologic Considerations

1. The classification of shock is a reflection of the underlying pathophysiology (Table 3-1).
   a. *Hypovolemic shock* results from a reduction in the circulating blood volume and preload, producing progressive dysfunction.

      There is an initial decreased preload due to capillary pooling and leakage accompanied by extrinsic and intrinsic loss of intravascular volume and decreased cardiac output. Arteriolar constriction results from increased afterload. The initial compensatory homeostasis is achieved at the expense of regional blood flow to the skin and muscles, and ultimately to the kidneys, mesentery, lungs, heart, and brain.
   b. *Cardiogenic shock* is accompanied by dysfunction of the heart causing decreased cardiac output from myocardial insufficiency or mechanical obstruction to flow into or out of the heart. Inadequate preload, with accompanying hypovolemia, capillary injury, vascular instability, and decreased cardiac output and tissue perfusion, all produce microcirculatory failure. Acidosis, hypoxemia, dysrhythmias, pulmonary embolism, pulmonary disease, and drug therapy may have an impact on the presentation. This may be the terminal event associated with other categories of shock.
   c. *Distributive or vasogenic shock* occurs with abnormal distribution of blood flow, initially resulting from acute arteriolar dilation and increased venous capacitance accompanied by decreased intravascular volume secondary to leaky capillaries. Septic shock often has an early hyperdynamic phase followed by a vasoconstrictive phase.

      Common agents responsible for anaphylactic shock include antigen extracts, antibiotics, insect stings (bee, wasp, yellow jacket), food, diagnostic agents, aspirin, narcotics, insulin, and inhaled allergens.
2. The degree of homeostatic compensation alters the presentation of a given type of shock. The relative compensation reflects the physiologic impact upon vascular resistance and cardiac output.
   a. *Compensated shock* results from the neuroendocrine reflex mediated by the baroreceptors in the heart and great vessels. These receptors stimulate the sympathetic nervous system in response to decreasing mean blood pressure. As fluid loss progresses, venous capacitance may decrease by 10–25%, fluid shifts from the interstitial to intravascular compartments, and arteriolar constriction increases. Tachycardia develops with increasing contractility of the heart and enhanced stroke volume.

Table 3-1. Etiologic Classification of Shock

Hypovolemia

1. Fluid and electrolyte loss
   a. Acute gastroenteritis (vomiting/diarrhea)
   b. Excessive sweating (cystic fibrosis)
   c. Renal pathology
2. Hemorrhage
   a. External: lacerations
   b. Internal: ruptured spleen or liver, vascular injury, fracture. In neonate: intracerebral/intraventricular hemorrhage
   c. Gastrointestinal: bleeding ulcer, ruptured viscus
3. Plasma loss
   a. Burn
   b. Inflammation or sepsis; leaky capillary syndrome
   c. Third spacing: intestinal obstruction, pancreatitis, peritonitis
4. Endocrine
   a. Adrenal insufficiency, adrenal-genital syndrome
   b. Diabetes mellitus
   c. Diabetes insipidus
   d. Hypothyroidism

Cardiogenic

1. Myocardial insufficiency
   a. Myocardial ischemia, infarction, rupture
   b. Structural lesion
   c. Cardiomyopathy: congestive, hypertropic, restrictive
   d. Dysrhythmia
   e. Drug intoxication
   f. Postcardiopulmonary bypass
   g. Myocardial depressant effect of shock
   h. Hypothermia
2. Filling or outflow obstruction
   a. Pericardial tamponade
   b. Pneumopericardium
   c. Valvular disease
   d. Tension pneumothorax
   e. Pulmonary embolism
   f. Congenital heart disease

Distributive

1. High or normal resistance (increased venous capacitance)
   a. Septic shock
   b. Anaphylaxis
2. Low resistance (vasodilation)
   a. CNS injury (spinal cord transection)

With progression, central venous pressure (CVP) decreases with accompanying redistribution of blood flow. Patients have orthostatic blood pressure (BP) changes (systolic BP decreases ≥ 15 mm Hg or pulse increases ≥ 20 beats/min) reflecting intravascular volume loss. Acidosis may be the most sensitive indicator of inadequate perfusion.

b. *Decompensated shock* occurs with progressive blood loss or myocardial dysfunction leading to exhaustion of compensatory mechanisms. This leads to lowered perfusion pressure, increased precapillary arteriolar resistance, and contraction of venous capacitance. Stagnation leads to anaerobic metabolism and release of proteolytic and vasoactive substances. Metabolic acidosis, respiratory compensation, and ultimately multisystem organ failure result.

Patients demonstrate hypotension, tachycardia, and multisystem failure with adult respiratory distress syndrome (ARDS), liver and pancreatic failure, gastrointestinal bleeding, coagulopathy with DIC, oliguria and renal failure, impaired mental status, acidosis, abnormal calcium and phosphorus homeostasis, and ongoing cellular damage.

Diagnostic Approach

1. *Historical data* is essential.
   - **a.** Nature and rapidity of progression, dizziness, mental status, and frequency and amount of urination reflecting the degree of compensation.
   - **b.** Preexisting and contributing conditions.
   - **c.** Specific aspects that delineate conditions contributing to shock.
2. *Physical examination* must be complete and should initially focus on hemodynamic stability after focusing on resuscitation.
   - **a.** Vital signs, specifically focusing on orthostatic changes in blood pressure and pulse, respiratory rate, temperature, and hydration status.
   - **b.** Capillary refill (normally < 2 sec).
   - **c.** Pulmonary and cardiac examination, looking for ronchi, rales, murmurs, and rubs.
   - **d.** Abdominal tenderness as well as blood in stool or gastric aspirate.
   - **e.** Mental status and alertness.
   - **f.** Specific findings related to primary condition.
3. *Diagnostic work-up*.
   - **a.** Laboratory.
     - **(1)** Chemistry: electrolytes, glucose, BUN, creatinine, liver function, calcium, phosphorus.
     - **(2)** Hematology: complete blood count (CBC), platelets, coagulation studies (prothrombin times, partial thromboplastin time; if DIC, fibrinogen, fibrin split products).
     - **(3)** ECG, chest x-ray film, echocardiogram.
     - **(4)** Urinalysis and urine output.
     - **(5)** Type and cross-match.
     - **(6)** Cultures of blood and urine.
     - **(7)** Other studies as indicated.
   - **b.** Therapeutic trial to assess the response to fluid bolus of 20 ml/kg of normal saline or lactated ringer's. This fluid challenge may be repeated if there is little or no response. If cardiogenic or distributive shock is suspected, pharmacologic response may need to be assessed.

Alert: All patients in shock require immediate assessment and stabilization of airway, breathing, and circulation. Following this stage, further evaluation and therapy should focus on other therapeutic maneuvers while assessing potential conditions contributing to the shock state.

Bibliography

American Academy of Pediatrics Committee on Drugs: Emergency drug doses in infants and children. Pediatrics 81:462, 1988.

Barkin RM, Rosen P: *Emergency pediatrics* (3rd ed.) St. Louis: C.V. Mosby, 1990.

Kanter RK, Zimmerman JJ, Strauss RH, et al.: Pediatric intravenous access. Amer J Dis Child 140:132, 1986.

Smith JAR and Normal JN: The fluid of choice for resuscitation of severe shock. Br J Surg 69:702, 1982.

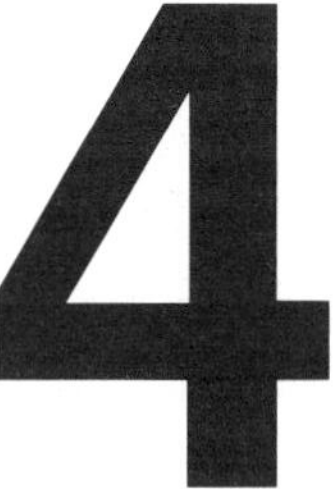

Fluid and Electrolyte Problems

Pediatric patients with fluid and electrolyte problems require an assessment of history and physical and laboratory data to determine the significance of any deficit. In addition, maintenance requirements and sources of abnormal loss must be understood.

Maintenance Fluids and Electrolytes

Maintenance fluid and electrolyte requirements primarily reflect daily water and electrolyte losses from the skin and the respiratory, urinary, and gastrointestinal tracts.

1. Fluid: urinary (60 ml/kg/24 hr), fecal (0–10 ml/kg/24 hr), and insensible (30 ml/kg/24 hr) losses amount to 100 ml/kg/24 hr in children to 10 kg and decreases on a per kilogram basis, thereafter.
   a. Insensible losses occur through the skin and respiratory tract. Water loss is affected by humidity, body temperature, respiratory rate, and ambient temperature. Fever increases insensible water loss by 7 ml/kg/24 hr for each degree rise in temperature above 37.2°C (99°F).
   b. Urinary losses reflect solute load and obligate excretion and urine concentration.
   c. Water requirements may be summarized:

Children < 10 kg	100 ml/kg/24 hr
Children 11–20 kg	1000 ml *plus* 50 ml/kg/24 hr for each kg above 10 kg
Children > 20 kg	1500 ml *plus* 20 ml/kg/24 hr for each kg above 20 kg
Adult	2000–2400 ml/24 hr

2. Electrolyte requirements reflect fluid losses and shifts. Sodium is primarily in the extracellular fluid (ECF) compartment, including intravascularly, while potassium is largely intracellular (ICF).
   Requirements of these cations include:

Sodium	3 mEq/kg/24 hr (adult: 80–100 mEq/24 hr)
Potassium	2 mEq/kg/24 hr (adult: 50 mEq/24 hr)

Electrolyte and Acid-Base Abnormalities

Sodium and potassium largely determine the distribution between the ECF and ICF spaces. This depends upon active transport of potassium into and sodium out of the cells by an energy-linked process.

Sodium

1. The concentration is affected by intake, total body water, and excretion through urine, sweat, and feces.

2. Hyponatremia.
   a. Clinical manifestations reflect the rapidity of progression, the severity, and the osmolality. Early signs include apathy, difficulty concentrating, and agitation, progressing to confusion, irritability, coma, and seizures. Nausea, vomiting, muscle weakness, myoclonus, and decreased deep tendon reflexes may be noted.
   b. Decreased total body water and relatively greater decrease in total body sodium. Examples: renal salt loss (diuretics, adrenal insufficiency, renal tubular acidosis), extrarenal salt loss (severe sweating, cystic fibrosis, GI losses, vomiting, diarrhea), third spacing (burns, peritonitis, pancreatitis).
   c. Increased total body water and normal body sodium. Examples: syndrome of inappropriate secretion of antidiuretic syndrome (SIADH) (pulmonary disease, CNS trauma, drugs such as hypoglycemic agents, antineoplastic drugs, tricyclics, and thiazide diuretics), hypothyroidism, severe potassium depletion, psychogenic water drinking.
   d. Increased total body water relatively greater than increased total body sodium. Examples: congestive heart failure, renal or hepatic failure, nephrosis, hypoproteinemia.
   e. Pseudohyponatremia. Examples: hyperglycemia (serum sodium decreases 1.6 mEq/L for each increment of 100 mg/dl rise in serum glucose), hyperproteinemia, hyperlipidemia.
3. Hypernatremia.
   a. Clinically, patients develop symptoms of altered mental status, irritability, seizures, and coma with associated skeletal muscle rigidity and hyperactive reflexes.
   b. Decreased total body water and normal total body sodium (dehydration). Examples: increased insensible or renal water loss, excessive solute loss (mannitol, urea), abnormal water loss (diarrhea), diabetes insipidus.
   c. Normal total body water and increased total body sodium. Examples: salt poisoning, rehydration with boiled milk, CNS disease affecting hypothalamus.

Potassium

1. Major cation of ICF. Only 1.5–2.0% of total body potassium is ECF.
2. Hypokalemia.
   a. Patients have muscle weakness, abdominal distension and decreased bowel sounds (ileus), impaired renal concentrating ability, and hypochloremic alkalosis. Delayed ventricular polarization may be noted with a relatively flat T wave on ECG. Dysrhythmias are more common in patients with myocarditis or those taking digoxin.
   b. Causes include excessive loss of potassium from the GI tract (diarrhea, vomiting, or NG suction), kidneys (diuretics, renal tubular acidosis), drug ingestion, and insulin or glucose therapy.
3. Hyperkalemia.
   a. Cardiac conduction abnormalities are common. A peaked T wave progresses to a widened QRS and ventricular dysrhythmias.
   b. Renal or metabolic disease may be causative, as well as acidosis or excessive intake. During metabolic acidosis, renal secretion of hydrogen ions is increased while that of potassium is decreased. For every 0.1 decrease in pH, serum potassium increases by about 0.5 mEq/L.

Acid-Base

1. Compensatory mechanisms usually occur with any primary acid-base abnormality. As noted, the primary problem is paralleled by compensating findings:

	pH	pCO_2	HCO_3^-
Metabolic acidosis	↓ *	↓	↓
Metabolic alkalosis	↑ *	↑	↑
Respiratory acidosis	↓	↑ *	↑
Respiratory alkalosis	↑	↓ *	↓

*Indicates primary abnormality

2. *Metabolic acidosis* is accompanied by compensatory tachypnea, sometimes associated with cardiac dysrhythmias and cellular dysfunction.
3. *Metabolic alkalosis* presents with muscle cramps, weakness, paresthesias, seizures, hyperreflexia, tetany, and dysrhythmias.

Diagnostic Approach to Dehydration

1. *Historically*, patients should be assessed to determine their hydration status.
   a. Hemodynamic instability focusing on dizziness, syncope, and mental status.
   b. Hydration by recording frequency, amount, and character of vomiting or diarrhea. Type and amount of intake must be assessed. Specific attention should be directed to the number of diapers, frequency and volume of urination, and any abnormal intake or output.
   c. Frequency of urination as a parameter of fluid balance can be assessed by determining the frequency of wet diapers and their relative weight or dampness. In older children, more specific questions about frequency can be asked.
   d. Preexisting cardiac, pulmonary, and renal disease should be defined.
2. *Physical examination* helps to determine fluid deficits.
   a. Assess vital signs and hemodynamic parameters. Adequacy of airway, breathing, and circulation must be demonstrated. Orthostatic blood pressure and pulse are particularly helpful. A decrease in blood pressure of 15 mm Hg or an increase of pulse of 20 beats/min after 2–3 minutes following changed position from lying to standing is considered significant.
   b. In a child with mild (2–5%) dehydration, slight decrease in mucosal membrane moisture and the relative dryness and prominence of the papillae of the tongue may be noted.
   c. As hydration status worsens, more specific findings are evident (Table 4-1).
   d. Evaluation of the patient in shock is presented in Chapter 3.
   e. Other components of the exam should focus on the source of dehydration.
   f. The type of dehydration reflecting serum osmolality is an important parameter in the moderately to severely dehydrated child to assess the etiology and degree of dehydration as well as therapeutic approaches (Table 4-2).

Table 4-1. Degree of Dehydration

	Mild (< 5%)	Moderate (10%)	Severe (> 10%)
Signs and symptoms			
Dry mucosal membrane	±	+	+
Reduced skin turgor	–	±	+
Sunken anterior fontanelle	–	+	+
Sunken eyeballs	–	+	+
Hyperpnea	–	±	+
Hypotension (orthostatic)	–	±	+
Tachycardia	–	+	+
Laboratory			
Urine			
Volume	Small	Oliguria	Oliguria/anuria
Specific gravity	≤ 1.020	> 1.030	> 1.035
Blood BUN	WNL*	Elevated	Very high

*Not usually indicated in mild dehydration
\+ present ± variable – absent

Table 4-2. Types of Dehydration

	Isotonic	Hypotonic	Hypertonic
Serum sodium (mEq/L)	130–150	< 130	> 150
Signs and symptoms			
Skin			
Color	gray	gray	gray
Temperature	cold	cold	cold
Turgor	poor	very poor	fair
Feel	dry	clammy	thick, doughy
Mucous membrane	dry	dry	parched
Sunken eyeballs	+	+	+
Depressed anterior fontanelle	+	+	+
Mental status	lethargic	coma/seizure	irritable/seizure
Increased pulse	+ +	+ +	+
Decreased BP	+ +	+ + +	+

3. *Diagnostic work-up* should include a number of studies in addition to those delineated above.

a. Laboratory.

(1) Chemistries: BUN, electrolytes, glucose. BUN is often elevated but with appropriate hydration will decrease by 50% over the first 24 hours. If this does not happen, consider other conditions such as hemolytic-uremic syndrome (HUS).

(2) Hematology: complete blood count to assess risk of infection.

(3) Urine specific gravity to confirm physical findings and monitor patient along with urine output.

b. Therapeutic trial in moderately to severely dehydrated patients may be useful in assessing the degree of dehydration and the response to initial therapy.

(1) D5W 0.9%NS or D5WLR should be given at 20 ml/kg (adult: 1–2 L) over 20 min. Glucose may be omitted from these solutions.

(2) If a poor response is noted, the initial infusion is followed by 10–20 ml/kg (adult: 0.5–1.0 L) over 20–30 min assuming normal renal and cardiac function. Optimally, this second infusion would not contain glucose.

(3) If the response is adequate, deficit and maintenance fluids should be administered (usually D5W 0.45%NS with 20 mEq KCl/L in isotonic dehydration). If response is poor, further evaluation and monitoring are usually required, focusing on renal function and possibly central venous pressure.

Alert: Dehydration requires assessment of the degree and type of fluid deficit and rapid correction while monitoring hemodynamic parameters.

Bibliography

American Academy of Pediatrics Committee on Nutrition: Use of oral fluid therapy and post-treatment feeding following enteritis in children in a developed country. Pediatrics 75:358, 1985.

Barkin RM, Rosen P: *Emergency Pediatrics* (3rd ed.) St. Louis: C.V. Mosby, 1990.

Pizarro D, Castillo B, Posada G, et al.: Efficacy comparison of oral rehydration solutions containing either 90 or 75 millimoles of sodium per liter. Pediatrics 79:190, 1987.

Winter, RW: *Principles of Pediatric Fluid Therapy* (2d ed.). Boston: Little, Brown, 1982.

5 Fever

The febrile child, particularly one under 2 years of age, presents unique challenges to the clinician because of the nonspecific nature of the history and findings. Over 10% of visits in this age group are for acute fevers, with the large majority of these being due to an infectious process.

The hypothalamus regulates temperature, establishing a set point based upon blood temperature. The set point may be increased by infection or malignancy and lowered by antipyretics. Heat is lost from the body by radiation, conduction, evaporation, and convection. These mechanisms for heat loss are limited in the presence of high environmental temperature, high humidity, and anhydrotic ectodermal dysplasia. (See also p. 259.)

Definition

Children are generally considered febrile when their rectal temperatures are 38.0°C (100.4°F) or higher. Oral temperatures greater than 37.6°C (99.7°F) are elevated. Although controversial, 37.3°C is defined as a febrile axillary value (Figure 5-1). Some diurnal variation exists in children over two years of age, with elevations of 1.0°C (1.8°F) being noted in the late afternoon or early evening. Newborns have some difficulty in thermoregulation, requiring a stable ambient temperature.

The *site* for temperature measurement must reflect proximity to major arteries, absence of inflammation, degree of precision required, safety, and insulation from external factors (such as drinking). *Rectal* temperatures provide precision, but obviously have the risk of rectal perforation and emotional trauma. *Axillary* temperatures are not practical in children under 4 years of age but are appropriate in thermostable environments or when absolute precision is not mandatory. Temperatures are not totally reliable in mildly febrile children (38–38.5°C). The *oral or sublinqual site* is useful in cooperative older children who do not have a rapid respiratory rate. The *tympanic membrane* has been used with great accuracy and reproducibility using new technology that is increasingly available.

As temperatures rise above 40°C, the risk of meningitis increases. However, fevers greater than 42°C (107.6°F) usually are not infectious in origin (e.g., they result from CNS involvement or heat stroke).

Etiologic Considerations

The vast majority of fevers in children are due to an acute infectious process. Infections may represent a local inflammatory process or a systematic infection. Less commonly, collagen vascular disease, neoplasm, or neurologic problems can be causative.

A fever of undetermined origin (FUO) is characterized by a fever of two weeks or more without localizing signs or a specific diagnosis. Although unusual in children, the differential considerations must include those delineated in Table 5-1. Careful documentation of the pattern, frequency, and height of temperature must be recorded over time.

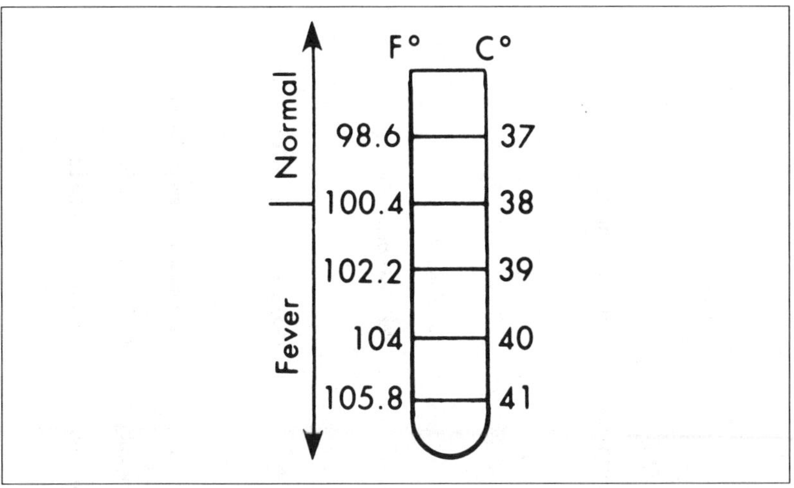

Figure 5-1. Conversion scale. (Reproduced by permission from Barkin RM and Rosen P: *Emergency Pediatrics: A Guide to Ambulatory Care* (3rd ed). St. Louis: C. V. Mosby, 1990.

Diagnostic Approach

A realistic approach is outlined in Figure 5-2 for the acutely febrile child under 2 years of age. Workup of more chronically ill children should incorporate evaluation of a number of other potential entities as indicated in Table 5-1. This often requires a CBC, ESR, cultures (blood, urine, CSF, and so on), appropriate x-rays, and other appropriate assessments.

1. *Historically*, parents usually report nonspecific observations related to behavior and associated signs and symptoms rather than those that permit an early focus on the involved system.
   a. Define alterations in behavior, activity, and eating habits.
   b. Determine if respiratory, gastrointestinal, musculoskeletal, and dermatologic findings have developed. Urinary tract and CNS symptoms are reflected in changes in behavior, such as irritability and lethargy.
   c. Exposures to children with similar complaints are important to note, as are recent events, such as DTP immunizations.
2. The *physical examination* to assess responsiveness must be done systematically. Focus on careful observation of the child at play and encourage the youngster to follow lights, bright objects, or a parent. Components of this overall assessment that are useful and reassuring include:
   a. Child looks and focuses on clinician and spontaneously explores the room.
   b. Child spontaneously makes sounds or talks in a playful manner.
   c. Child plays and reaches for objects.
   d. Child smiles and interacts with parent or practitioner.
   e. Child quiets easily when held by parent.
3. *Early antipyretic therapy* is imperative in facilitating observation. Many children who initially are irritable and disinterested in their environment will improve markedly with aggressive antipyretic management. Acetaminophen (15 mg/kg/dose PO or PR) should be administered to all children with temperatures greater than 38.5°C (101.3°F) on *arrival* in the clinic or ED to ensure optimal observation by reducing temperature and permitting a more accurate assessment of the child. Children with temperatures greater than 39.5°C (103°F) should also be sponged with tepid water. The response to antipyretics does not predict the prevalence of bacteremia.

Table 5-1. Fever: Etiologic Considerations

Condition	Diagnostic Findings	Ancillary Data	Comments
Infection/Inflammation			
Respiratory (see Chap. 44 and 46)			
URI Otitis media Pharyngitis Pneumonia Exanthems	Variable respiratory findings	CBC, throat culture, chest x-ray	Often self-limited
Gastrointestinal (see Chap. 23 and 26)			
Gastroenteritis Ova and parasites	Vomiting, diarrhea	Stool polys, CBC	Variable fever
Appendicitis, peritonitis	Abdominal tenderness, vomiting, poor intake	WBC elevated, UA normal	Variable other pathology
Hepatitis	Liver tenderness, vomiting	Liver function	
Cholangitis		Ultrasound	
Urinary tract (Chap. 40)	Burning, dysuria, frequency	Urinalysis, culture	Common in young girl
Central nervous system (Chap. 32)			
Meningitis Encephalitis	Altered mental status	CSF, CT scan	
Bacteremia	Children $<$ 24 mo, multiple foci, fever $>$ 39.4°C	WBC $>$ 15,000/mm^3; blood culture, urinalysis, chest x-ray	Presumptive therapy, follow-up
Osteomyelitis (Chap. 38 and 39)	Bony tenderness	WBC, ESR elevated, x-ray, blood culture	Prolonged antibiotics
Abcess Lung Abdominal, pelvic Perinephric	Reflects location	WBC, radiographs, aspiration	Multiple potential sites

Trauma/Environment			
CNS trauma (Chap. 47)	Altered mental status	CT scan	Altered set point
Hyperthermia	Altered fluid status, mentation	Electrolytes	
Congenital			
Ectodermal dysplasia	Abnormal sweating, skin	Electrolytes	Inability to sweat
Sickle cell disease	Crisis, abdominal pain, fever	Hct, reticulocyte count	
Congenital dysautonomia			
Malignant hyperthermia	Muscle contraction, tachypnea, acidosis		Halogenated inhalation agent
Collagen-Vascular			
Juvenile rheumatoid arthritis (Chap. 38)	Variable presentation, prognosis	WBC, ESR, ANA	
Inflammatory bowel disease		WBC, ESR, GI contrast study	
Neoplasm	Variable presentation		
Intoxication			
Drug fever	Onset of fever with specific drug	Withdrawal drug	
Immunizations (DTP)			
Salicylate			
Miscellaneous			
Dehydration (Chap. 4)	Evidence of fluid deficit	Electrolytes, urinalysis	Fluid replacement
Transfusion reaction	Serum sickness-like reaction		
Hyperthyroidism			

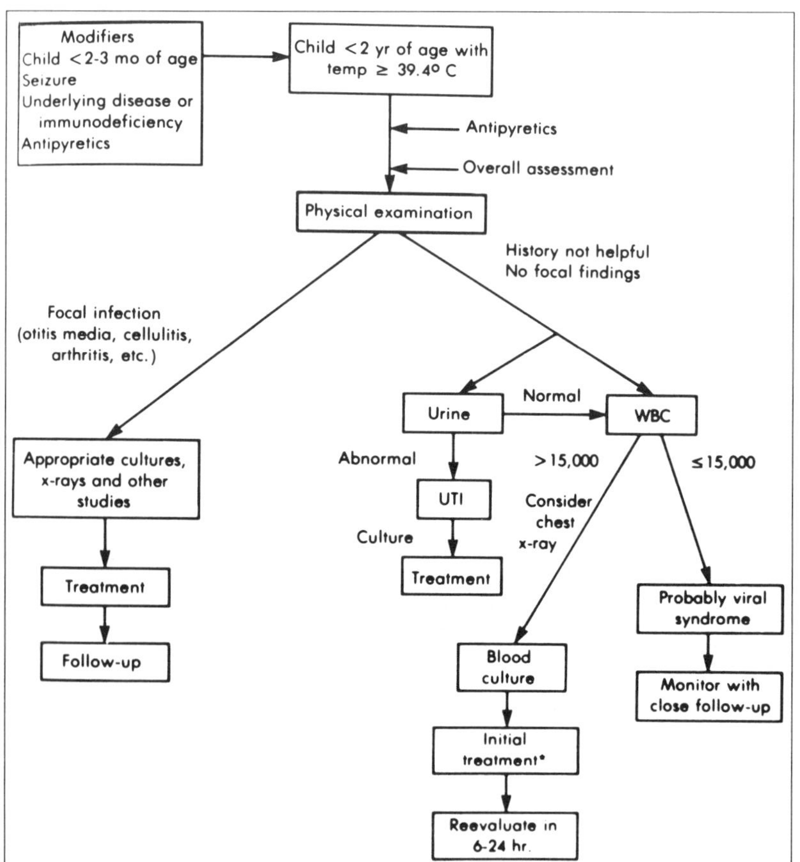

Figure 5-2. Evaluation of the febrile child under 2 yr. *Ceftriaxone 50 mg/kg/dose IM/IV; ampicillin 50–75 mg/kg/dose IM/IV; or amoxicillin 70–75 mg/kg/24 hr q 8 hr PO pending cultures. (Reproduced by permission from Barkin RM and Rosen P: *Emergency Pediatrics: A Guide to Ambulatory Care* (3rd ed). St. Louis: C. V. Mosby, 1990.

While the child is distracted with play objects, obvious physical abnormalities should be noted and examined.

a. Hemodynamic instability, petechiae, and purpura require emergent intervention.

b. Limitation of limb movement, rashes, and points of tenderness or pain should be defined.

c. The chest, heart, and abdomen require a gentle hand and patience. Tachypnea disproportionate to fever must be carefully evaluated, usually through a chest x-ray.

d. A full examination of ears, throat, neck, and so on.

Infants Under Two to Three Months of Age

A more extensive evaluation is required. The history is rarely more specific than the triad of fever, irritability, and poor feeding, and the physical examination may fail to reveal specific focal findings despite the presence of systemic infections, which may be enteric, as well as the more common organisms infecting older children. Children under 3 months with a temperature greater than 38.5°C have a greater than 20-fold risk of having a serious infection than do older children with a similar temperature.

Prospective studies have demonstrated that clinical judgment is *not* useful in the assessment of the young febrile infant. There are no clear factors that are sensitive or specific to rely on in decision making. However, factors that have been most consistently associated with bacterial disease include: age under 1 month, history of lethargy, no contact with an ill person, breastfeeding, PMN count greater than 10,000/mm^3, and band count over 500/mm^3. *No laboratory or historical factors should be used to exclude underlying bacterial infection.*

Children under 2–3 months with temperatures over 38°C (rectal) usually require blood cultures, urinalysis, and lumbar puncture unless they look remarkably well and follow-up is absolute. Infants should generally be admitted and started on broad spectrum antibiotics.

Immunocompromised Children

Children with a history of recurrent serious bacterial infection should be evaluated for immunodeficiency. Children undergoing cancer chemotherapy or with a history of asplenia (e.g., congenital, trauma) are obviously at risk. Those with sickle cell disease have a 400-fold increased risk of pneumococcal septicemia if under 5 years of age and a 4-fold risk of *H. influenzae* septicemia if under 9 years of age. Such children require an aggressive and anticipatory approach to potential infections.

Occult Bacteremia

Although bacteremia occurs in association with a host of clinical entities, including meningitis, arthritis, epiglottitis, cellulitis, pneumonia, and kidney infections, about 6% of febrile patients without a defined focus have positive blood cultures. Occult bacteremia is a significant problem in children, the high risk group being defined as:

Age: ≤ 24 mo
Fever: ≥ 39.4°C (102.9°F)
WBC: ≥ 15,000 mm^3 (differential does not increase prognostic value)
ESR: ≥ 30 mm/hr (difficult to use because of the length of time required to obtain result)

It is essential to evaluate such children carefully to be certain that there is no underlying disease such as pneumonia or meningitis. There is no conclusive evidence that performing a lumbar puncture on a bacteremic child significantly increases the risk of subsequently developing meningitis.

Organisms that are frequently cultured include *Steptococcus pneumoniae* and *Haemophilus influenzae*. *Staphylococcus aureus* and *Neisseria meningitidis* are less common pathogens. Children under 2 or 3 months of age may also develop infections caused by *Escherichia coli* and *Listeria monocytogenes* and therefore require broader antibiotic coverage.

Special aspects of the evaluation of the acutely ill child to consider (Figure 5-2):

1. Early antipyretic therapy will facilitate assessment. Previous antipyretic therapy requires a lower temperature threshold for initiating laboratory evaluation.
2. Underlying cardiac, pulmonary, neurologic, and immunodeficiency (e.g., sickle cell, neoplasm, steroids) diseases require early evaluation and treatment, regardless of age and the height of fever.
3. Meningitis must be considered in any febrile child who has a seizure. Children 12 months of age and younger should have a spinal tap (Table 32-2). A temperature of 41.1°C or higher is associated with a 10% incidence of meningitis in children under 2 years of age.
4. Children with fever and petechiae may have a viral illness, Rocky Mountain spotted fever, or invasive bacterial disease. Rapid intervention is required. Children with fever and petechiae and a normal LP and WBC count (normal absolute neutrophil and band count), and a temperature of less than 40°C have a reduced risk of having a bacterial infection.
5. If the temperature in a child younger than 6 months has been present for less than 24

hours, the child looks well on the basis of overall assessment, and no helpful history is detected, close follow-up for 6–12 hours may substitute for laboratory evaluation at the time of the first encounter. If the temperature remains elevated above 39.4°C at the follow-up appointment, evaluation should proceed.

6. Children with WBC greater than 15,000 mm^3 from whom blood cultures have been obtained may be treated with antibiotics with the potential to reduce complications. Alternative regimens include amoxicillin 50–100 mg/kg/24 hr PO, cefaclor 40 mg/kg/24 hr PO, ampicillin 50 mg/kg/dose IM or IV, or ceftriaxone 50 mg/kg/24 hr (or other third generation cephalosporin) IM or IV.

7. *Follow-up is essential*, usually in 6–12 hours, depending upon clinical and logistical constraints.

a. If the cultures remain negative, antibiotics may be stopped after 48 hours unless there was a specific focus initially or one develops. Follow-up until resolution of the illness is necessary.

b. If the culture is positive, thereby documenting bacteremia, reexamination of the patient should generally determine treatment.

(1) A patient who has a totally normal examination should continue taking high-dose antibiotics as an outpatient if daily contact can be maintained or as an inpatient if compliance is questionable. A total 10-day course is necessary. Most patients who have been treated initially will be improved on follow-up, but this does not preclude the importance of continuing antibiotics. *N. meningitidis* may require parenteral treatment.

(2) Febrile or toxic patients or patients who develop a focus should be admitted for intravenous antibiotics and further evaluation. A total course of 10 days is necessary.

Alert: The acutely ill child must be evaluated to exclude serious underlying disease, while focusing on differential considerations. Prolonged fevers may require a more extensive evaluation.

Bibliography

Bell LM: Management of the febrile child under 2 years of age. In Barkin RM (ed): *The Emergently Ill Child*. Rockville: Aspen Publishers, 1987.

Berkowitz CD: Assessment and management of the febrile infant under 2 months of age. In Barkin RM (ed): *The Emergently Ill Child*. Rockville: Aspen Publishers, 1987.

Jaffe DM, Tanz RR, Davis AT, et al.: Antibiotic administration to treat possible occult bacteremia in febrile children. New Eng. J. Med. 317: 1175, 1987.

Lui CH, Lehan C, Speer, ME, et al.: Early detection of bacteremia in an outpatient clinic. Pediatrics 75: 827, 1985.

Powell KR, Mawhorter SD: Outpatient treatment of serious infections in infants and children with ceftriaxone. J. Pediatr. 610: 898, 1987.

Yamamoto LT, Wigder HN, Fligner DJ, et al.: Relationship of bacteremia to antipyretic therapy in febrile children. Pediatr. Emerg. Care 3:223, 1987.

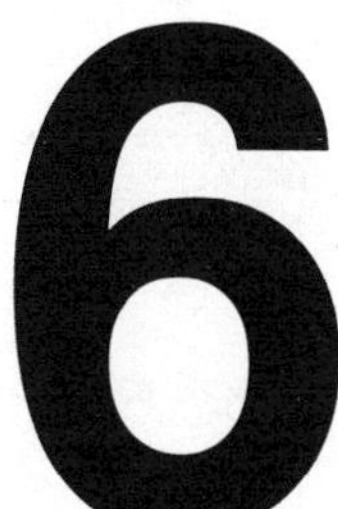

Failure to Thrive

Children who deviate from their normal growth curve or are two standard deviations below the age-specific mean for other children are considered to be failing to thrive (Appendix B). There must be an abnormal pattern or velocity of growth; it is not enough that a child is small, has always been small, and is growing consistently along his or her growth curve.

Parameters that may be useful in assessing growth patterns include:

1. Weight. Birth weight (average): 3.3 kg (7 lb 5 oz).
   A newborn has usually regained birth weight by 10 days of age and gains 30 g (1 oz)/day for the first 1–2 months.
   5 months: birth weight doubled.
   12 months: birth weight tripled.
2. Length. Birth length (average): 50 cm (20 in).
   12 months: birth length doubled.
3. Head Circumference (FOC – frontal occipital circumference). Birth head circumference (average): 35 cm (14 in). Head circumference grows 1 cm/month during the first 9 months of age.
   12 months: 47 cm (19 in).

Etiologic Considerations

Children who are failing to thrive generally have a nonorganic etiology, reflecting a variety of environmental, dietary, social, and parental issues. However, specific conditions should be considered in the evaluation (Table 6-1).

Several general patterns may be observed in assessing the pattern along a child's specific growth curve:

1. Primary *weight* fall off is generally a reflection of abnormal caloric intake, absorption, or loss.
2. Primary *height* fall off with minimal weight and FOC change is generally endocrinologic in origin.
3. Primary *head circumference* fall off without significant change in weight or height is usually due to CNS disease.

Diagnostic Approach

1. The *history* provides a basis for evaluating the pattern of growth and potential contributing conditions.
   a. Specific parameters of weight, height, and head circumference plotted on a standard growth curve (Appendix B), looking for a pattern and deviations.
   b. Specific environmental, physical, or other changes corresponding to change in pattern. Family growth pattern of sibling and parents.
   c. Observation of feeding, bonding, parenting, and so on.

Table 6-1. Failure to Thrive: Etiologic Considerations

Condition	Diagnostic Findings	Comments
Infection/Inflammation		
Urinary tract infection (Chap. 40)	Dysuria, frequency, burning, low grade fever; urinalysis and culture	May be asymptomatic
Respiratory infection (Chap. 46)	Prolonged or recurrent otitis media, sinusitis, pneumonia	Chronic infection
Gastroenteritis (Chap. 23 and 26)	Vomiting, diarrhea; stool leukocytes, culture, ELISA for rotavirus; dietary manipulation may be essential	May be post-infectious or acutely due to viral, bacterial, parasite
Hepatitis	Jaundice, malaise, vomiting; abnormal liver function	Acute or chronic
Congenital		
Cleft lip, palate	Often associated with feeding problems; responds to special nipples and careful feeding	Exclude associated anomaly
Gastroesophageal reflux (Chap. 26)	Vomiting or spitting; rarely apnea, recurrent wheezing, cough, pneumonitis, aspiration	May have associated hiatal hernia
Cystic fibrosis	Recurrent pulmonary and GI disease; stool: steatorrhea; sweat test	
Vitamin D resistance	Multiple fractures; vitamin D resistance, deficiency	
Congenital heart disease	Shortness of breath, feeding difficulty	May also be acquired
Allergic		
Asthma	Recurrent pneumonia, wheezing, shortness of breath; cough may be only finding	Other chronic pulmonary disease should be considered
Food sensitivity or intolerance	Diarrhea, vomiting, abdominal pain; variable hematest positive	Exclusion diet may be diagnostic

Endocrine/Metabolic		
Thyroid Hyper-/hypo	Variable findings; poor weight, height growth; thyroid function tests	
Hypopituitarism	Poor growth; sexual, thyroid dysfunction; hypoglycemia	Delayed onset in first 1–2 years of life
Adrenal Hyper-/hypo	Variable findings; hypo: lethargy, fatigue, increased pigmentation; hyper: Cushing's syndrome	
Diabetes mellitus	Polyuria, polydipsia; hyperglycemia; ketosis, acidosis	
Inborn error of metabolism	Multiple presentations	Galactosemia, storage disease
Renal tubular acidosis	Renal acidosis, hyperchloremic acidosis	Acquired or congenital; renal disease
Other		
Familial/environmental	Good initial velocity of growth; fall off in weight disproportionate; history, physical unremarkable; laboratory normal, bone age equal to chronologic age	Evaluate parenting pattern; may be due to knowledge, stress, neglect
Caloric deprivation	Insufficient caloric intake	May be feeding technique, insufficient calories, malabsorption (celiac, infection, intolerance); may be due to inadequate breast milk (newborn)
Constitutional	Small with normal velocity of growth; similar to parents, sibs pattern	
Neurologic	Abnormal cerebral function, exam	Acquired or congenital
Neoplasm	Variable presentation	
Collagen vascular disease		Juvenile rheumatoid arthritis, SLE, inflammatory bowel disease
Iron deficiency anemia (Chap. 29)	Malaise, anemia (hypochromic, microcytic); CBC and indices	

   d. Clinical signs of deprivation, including poor hygiene, cradle cap, diaper rash, and impetigo.
   e. Insidious or chronic findings associated with recurrent illness. Recent onset of infection, diarrhea, or vomiting.
2. On *physical examination*, often no abnormalities are detected, but a concerted search is obligatory.
   a. Growth parameters, blood pressure, pulse, and respiratory rate and pattern. Evaluate relative percentiles for each measurement. A history of similar patterns may be helpful.
   b. Complete physical examination looking for stigmata of underlying disease.
   c. Observation of feeding and parental bonding. Consider whether there has been any environmental or psychosocial disruption of the family including divorce, alcoholism, or prior abuse.
3. *Diagnostic work-up* should include some general screening measures and specific additional evaluation as indicated by the history and physical examination.
   a. Laboratory screens include:
      (1) Chemistries: Glucose, electrolytes.
      (2) Hematology: CBC, ESR, urinalysis.
      (3) Urine culture to exclude infection.
      (4) Radiologic evaluation should initially include a bone age.
   b. Therapeutic trial of child with primary weight loss of close observation and concerted attempts by knowledgeable and supportive personnel to maximize caloric intake and watch subsequent growth pattern either on an inpatient or outpatient basis depending upon specific circumstances.

Alert: Although nonorganic causes are most typical, treatable conditions should be excluded. Support, reassurance, and close monitoring are essential.

Bibliography

Berwick D: Nonorganic failure-to-thrive. Pediatr Rev 1:265, 1980.

Hufton I and Oates R: Nonorganic failure to thrive: a long-term follow-up. Pediatrics 59:73, 1977.

Rosenn D, Loeb L, Jura M: Differentiation of organic from nonorganic failure to thrive syndrome in infancy. Pediatrics 66:698, 1980.

Sills R: Failure to thrive: the role of clinical and laboratory evaluation. Am J Dis Child 132:967, 1978.

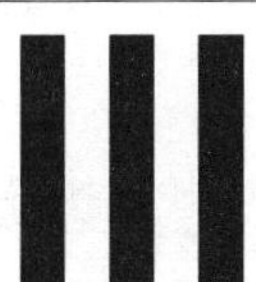

Behavioral Problems

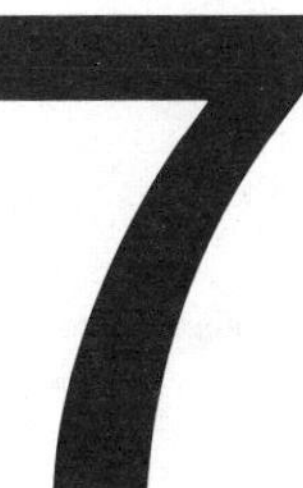

Encopresis

A child's inability to control bowel movements after 4 years of age is problematic. Children with encopresis often have overflow diarrhea (often water loss) and do not sense the need to have a bowel movement. They may feel isolated and unique, they may fear exposure, and they often develop behavioral problems. (See also p. 248.)

Etiologic Considerations

Factors that precipitate encopresis in children may be anatomical or functional, often reflecting stress upon the child.

1. Infants: constipation, congenital anorectal or acquired anorectal (fissure) problems, and parental overconcern with toilet training.
2. Toddlers: overemphasis on toilet training, family stress, painful defecation.
3. Children: prolonged gastroenteritis, psychosocial stresses at home or school, painful defecation, retardation, hyperactivity.

Rarely, organic conditions such as central nervous system disorders (may have accompanying urinary incontinence), hypothyroidism, calcium abnormalities, and aganglionic megacolon may be contributory.

Diagnostic Approach

1. *History* should focus on developmental and behavioral issues.
   a. Evaluate psychosocial adaptation and response to stress. Determine underlying psychiatric disease and developmental status (See Chap. 1).
   b. Determine response to previous therapy and therapeutic trials.
2. *Physical examination*.
   a. Exclude gastrointestinal, neurological, and endocrine pathology.
   b. Stool retention (see Chap. 22 on constipation) may be noted on rectal examination.
3. *Diagnostic approach*.
   a. Laboratory evaluation is rarely needed but may include specific tests to exclude underlying pathology. Girls with encopresis often have recurrent urinary tract infections due to ascending contamination and should have a urinalysis and culture.
   b. Therapeutic trial. The most important focus of the evaluation should be to assess the child's behavior and mental health with appropriate referral, often in combination with aggressive management of constipation (see Chap. 22).

Alert: Encopresis may be the function of, or secondary to, behavioral problems. Physiologic and psychologic problems must be dealt with concurrently.

Bibliography

Hatch T: Encopresis and constipation in children. Pediatr Clin North Am 35:257, 1988.

Rappaport L, et al.: Locus of control as prediction of compliance and outcome in treatment of encopresis. J Pediatr 109:1061, 1986.

8 Enuresis

Girls normally have bladder control after 5 years of age; boys may not have control until 6 years of age. Daytime or diurnal enuresis occurs first. Nocturnal enuresis exists in approximately 15% of all 5-year-olds, 7% of 8-year-olds, and 3% of 12-year-olds. Children who have never been consistently dry are considered to have primary enuresis while those who were previously dry for 3–6 months are termed secondary enuretics.

Etiologic Considerations

Delays in neuromuscular maturation and a smaller functional bladder are commonly causative of primary enuresis.

Anatomical abnormalities of the genitourinary and nervous systems may also be contributory. Obstructive lesions of the distal outflow tract including posterior urethral valves, diverticulum of the anterior urethra, neurologically abnormal bladder function (meningomyelocele, sacral agenesis, neurogenic bladder, seizures) as well as urinary tract infections (Chap. 40) may be present.

Psychologic problems and environmental stress have both been implicated in secondary enuresis. Stress incontinence from excessive Valsalva's maneuver or coughing may occur. Resistance to toilet training is often associated with enuresis. Diabetes mellitus, diabetes insipidus, sickle cell trait, renal tubular disease, and diuretics have been infrequent causes.

Diagnostic Approach

1. *History* should define the type and pattern of enuresis.
   a. Pattern of bedwetting (night versus day; primary versus secondary).
   b. Response to therapeutic trials including waking child up, restricting fluid, positive reinforcement.
   c. Evidence of other diseases.
   d. Stress and environmental changes.
   e. Psychologic and developmental status of child. Presence of encopresis.
2. *Physical examination* is typically normal but should include a specific evaluation of the genitourinary and central nervous systems.
3. *Diagnostic approach.*
   a. Laboratory evaluation should be conducted as appropriate but at a minimum must include a urinalysis and urine culture.
   b. Radiologic studies should be done if the urine is abnormal. Assessment should include an ultrasound, voiding cystourethrogram (VCUG), or intravenous pyelogram (IVP).
   c. Therapeutic trial may include reviewing the response to management. A positive, upbeat approach is most useful, providing positive responses for the child while attempting to minimize stress and optimizing praise. Rarely are pharmacologic agents required.

Alert: Bedwetting is commonly part of normal development, but if prolonged past the normal age parameters, evaluation may be appropriate.

Bibliography

Doleys D and Dolce J: Toilet training and enuresis. Pediatr Clin North Am 29:297, 1982.

Moffatt MEK, Katoa C, Pless IB: Improvements in self-concept after treatment of nocturnal enuresis: randomized controlled trial. J Pediatr 110:647, 1987.

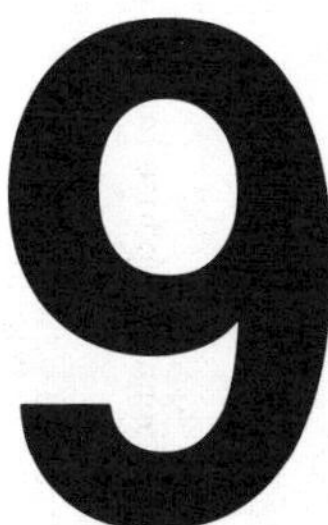

Irritability

Irritability in children is truly a relative term, reflecting changes in behavior that produce an unusual pattern for a given youngster. Changes in a child's usual personality are best gauged by the parents and are often a reflection of illness or stress in the child or his or her family. If frustration and turmoil exist, it is essential that this be recognized so that parents can be supported. Acute onset of irritability requires specific attention to delineating treatable or emergent conditions.

Most children have some period of the day when they are most irritable, usually toward the evening. In infants, when this progresses, it is referred to as colic and occurs in up to 10% of children. When present, it usually begins at 2–3 weeks of age and may continue through 10–12 weeks. The quieting response to soothing, rhythmical activities such as rocking are reassuring. Irritability from teething is often noted as the child gets older. (See also p. 247.)

Etiologic Considerations

Conditions leading to acute or chronic irritability may stem from a variety of processes (Table 9-1).

Diagnostic Approach

1. *History* should focus on the pattern of irritability.
   a. Time and duration, frequency, and factors to reduce or exacerbate irritability. Response to being consoled, feeding, or rocking should be sought. Factors that bring on irritability should be defined, such as loud noises, hunger, wet diapers, or searching for attention. Repetitive nature of the irritability.
   b. Preexisting and underlying conditions.
   c. Exclude potential contributing causes including trauma, medication, infection, congenital anomalies, and metabolic abnormalities. This is particularly important in children with acute behavioral changes.
   d. Evaluate the nature of parent-child bonding.
   e. If the child is teething, evaluate response to local therapy.
2. *Physical examination* should generally determine that the child is well, having no specific problems and a normal physical.
   a. Exclude recent trauma, congenital problems, infection, and evidence of metabolic abnormalities. It is essential to assure that no acute condition exists.
   b. Determine status of tooth eruption.
3. *Diagnostic work-up* is usually not required unless there are specific indications of an abnormality. If appropriate, laboratory evaluation should focus on excluding specific entities. Generally, reassurance and frequent contact and follow-up replace an extensive work-up (Table 9-1).

   Alert: Irritability is most commonly caused by colic in infants and requires a great deal of support for the parents. If there is any suspicion of underlying pathology, an

Table 9-1. Irritability: Etiologic Considerations

Condition	Diagnostic Findings	Comments
Infection		
Respiratory (Chap. 44)	Rhinorrhea, fever, ear pain, decreased activity, variable toxicity	Irritability decreases with antipyretics; must rule out other pathology
Urinary tract (Chap. 40)	Fever, dysuria, frequency, burning	Irritability decreases in 24 hours with antibiotics
Meningitis Encephalitis	Fever, anorexia, changed mental status, lethargy, variable stiff neck, headache	Important consideration in irritable child; may co-exist with other infections
Other	Associated signs and symptoms	
Trauma		
Foreign body, fracture, tourniquet	Local tenderness, swelling; thread around digit, penis	Splinter, hairline fracture, contusion
Subdural/epidural hematoma	History of head trauma, impaired mental status	Acute or chronic; CT scan
Corneal abrasion	May not have history; positive fluorescein examination	
Intoxication		
Sympathomimetics	Irritability as primary or side effect	Ephedrine, aminophylline, amphetamines, etc.
Lead	Weakness, weight loss, headache, abdominal pain, seizures	Decreasing in frequency
Deficiency		
Iron deficiency anemia	Pallor, learning deficit, poor diet, anorexia	Peaks at 9 and 18 months; diet insufficient; response to iron (Chap. 29)
Malnutrition	Wasted, distended abdomen	Neglect or poverty, scurvy, celiac disease
Endocrine/Metabolic (Chap. 4 and 31)		
Hypo-/hypernatremia	Dehydration, edema, seizure	Multiple etiologies

Hypo-/hypercalcemia	Tetany, seizure, diarrhea, abdominal pain, constipation, nephrocalcinosis	Multiple etiologies
Hypokalemia	Muscle weakness, ileus	Multiple etiologies
Hypoglycemia	Sweating, tachycardia, weakness, tachypnea, anxiety, decreased mental status	Multiple etiologies
Vascular		
Congenital heart disease	Cyanosis, other findings	Often cyanotic, congestive heart failure
Congestive heart failure	Tachypnea, tachycardia, rales, pulmonary edema	Multiple etiologies; insidious or rapid onset
Paroxysmal atrial tachycardia (Chap. 11)	Tachycardia > 200 beats/min, restless, variable decompensation	Multiple etiologies
Miscellaneous		
Colic (Chap. 20)	Episodic, intense, persistent crying in otherwise healthy child; usually late afternoon	Usually between 2–12 weeks of age
Teething	Irritated, swollen gums; does not cause high fever, significant diarrhea	Soothe with teething ring, wet wash cloth to chew on, etc.
Parental anxiety	Anxious, insecure parents; overly responsive to irritable, well child	Inconsistent parenting, unstable, changing environment

aggressive evaluation should be undertaken. Acute onset of irritability requires attention to excluding infectious, traumatic, or metabolic conditions.

Bibliography

Harley, LM: Fussing and crying in young infants. Clin Pediatr 8:138, 1969.

Honig PJ: Teething: are today's pediatricians using yesterday's notions? J Pediatr 87:415, 1975.

Zuckerman B, Stevenson J, and Bailey V: Sleep problems in early childhood: continuities, predictive factors, and behavior correlates. Pediatrics 80:664, 1987.

IV Cardiovascular Problems

10 Chest Pain

Chest pain in children occasionally suggests a serious underlying condition but is rarely as significant as this symptom is in adults. Somatic and visceral structures share sensory pathways. Visceral pathology may have somatic manifestations from T1–T6. Abdominal pathology may cause chest pain; posterior and lateral sections of the diaphragm are innervated by intercostal nerves and may be referred to the lower thorax and abdomen. The central and anterior portions are referred to the shoulder and neck regions.

Etiologic Considerations

Disorders from chest wall trauma account for nearly half of the cases, including costochondritis, discomfort from coughing, and muscle strain or trauma. Approximately one-third are idiopathic in origin while the remainder are considered functional. Very rarely are significant cardiac, vascular, or pulmonary disorders underlying conditions (Table 10-1).

Diagnostic Approach

1. *History* must focus on a number of components.
   a. The pain should be characterized with respect to onset and progression, character, severity, location, radiation, relationship to position, breathing, reproducibility, and factors that improve or exacerbate the intensity.
   b. Focus on past lung or heart problems, family history of heart, vascular, or pulmonary disease, medications (particularly oral birth control pills), coagulopathies, sickle cell disease, and other predisposing conditions.
   c. Recent trauma is commonly reported as is exacerbation with movement, coughing, or swallowing.
   d. Associated problems such as syncope, shortness of breath and exercise intolerance should be investigated.

      Pleurisy is often associated with underlying inflammatory disease. The pain is sharp in intensity, well localized over the involved area, perceived as superficial with a sensation of "catching"; pain is accentuated by deep breathing, coughing, and arm movement. Tenderness may be localized.
2. *Physical examination* must carefully focus on the chest, heart, and abdomen.
   a. Careful assessment of hemodynamic instability. Blood pressure, regularity of rhythm, and abnormalities of pulse should be determined.
   b. Auscultation, percussion, and palpatation. Pleural or pericardial friction rubs should be excluded.
   c. Reproducibility of the pain with movement or palpation is an important finding. A specific examination of the chest wall should be done.
3. *Diagnostic work-up* should include at least a chest x-ray. An ECG, ABG/oximetry, echocardiography, cardiac enzymes, V/Q scan, and abdominal work-up may be needed for specific indications (Table 10-1).

Table 10-1. Chest Pain: Etiologic Considerations

Condition	Diagnostic Findings	Ancillary Data	Comments
Infection/Inflammation			
Pneumonia	Cough, fever, tachypnea, variable distress, pleurisy	Chest x-ray, CBC, ABG/oximetry	Bacterial, viral origin
Pleurodynia	Sharp, stabbing pain; unilateral or bilateral; may recur	Chest x-ray	Coxsackie virus
Asthma	Wheezing, respiratory distress, coughing	Chest x-ray, ABG/oximetry	Pain due to muscle strain, pneumothorax, anxiety
Pericarditis	Sudden onset sharp substernal pain over precordium, epigastrium, or entire thorax; pain accentuated by deep breathing, cough, movement	Chest x-ray, ECG	Usually viral; may be associated with myocarditis or collagen-vascular disease
Esophagitis	Substernal pain, vomiting; evidence reflux; position and antacid influence	Also associated with hiatal hernia, foreign body, fear	
Abdominal pathology	Referred pain; symptoms related to pathology (peritonitis, hepatitis, appendicitis, etc.)	As indicated by pathology	
Trauma			
Muscle strain	Point tenderness, pain reproducible with pressure or activity	Chest x-ray	May be caused by coughing, new activity
Trauma to chest or abdomen	History trauma, local tenderness, referred pain, variably stable	Chest x-ray	Exclude pneumothorax, surgical problem
Vascular			
Angina, infarct, ischemia	Crushing, sharp pain over left chest with radiation to arm, neck, jaw; shortness of breath; cardiac decompensation	Chest x-ray, ECG	Sickle cell, pulmonary/aortic stenosis, dysrhythmia, etc.

Pulmonary embolism	Dyspnea, tachypnea, hemoptysis	V/Q scan, ECG, chest x-ray	Hyperventilation may simulate
Dissecting aortic aneurysm	Chest, abdominal, back pain; asymmetric pulses	Chest x-ray, ECG, CT or ultrasound	May be life threatening; Marfan, Ehler-Danlos
Mitral valve prolapse	Sharp of dull left pain; midsystolic click	Chest x-ray, ECG, echocardiogram	Usually asymptomatic
Psychogenic			
Functional	Acute stress, inconsistent	Chest x-ray	Evaluate environment
Hyperventilation	Tachypnea, weakness, tingling, dyspnea	Chest x-ray	May mimic pulmonary embolism
Other			
Idiopathic	Variable presentation	Chest x-ray	Most common
Pneumothorax	Acute onset pain, variable tachypnea	Chest x-ray	May be spontaneous

Alert: Chest pain is commonly associated with trauma. If vital signs are abnormal or there is a history of contributory predisposing conditions, significant underlying cardiac or pulmonary disease should be considered.

Bibliography

Asnes RS, Santulli R, Bemporad JR: Psychogenic chest pain in children. Clin Pediatr 20:788, 1981.

Brenner JI, Ringel RE, and Berman MA: Cardiologic perspective of chest pain in childhood: a referral problem. Pediatr Clin North Am 31:1241, 1984.

Driscoll DJ, Glicklich LB, and Gallen WJ: Chest pain in children: a prospective study. Pediatrics 57:648, 1976.

Pantell RH and Goodman BW: Adolescent chest pain: a prospective study. Pediatrics 71:881, 1983.

Selbst S, et al.: Pediatric chest pain: a prospective study. Pediatrics 82:319, 1988.

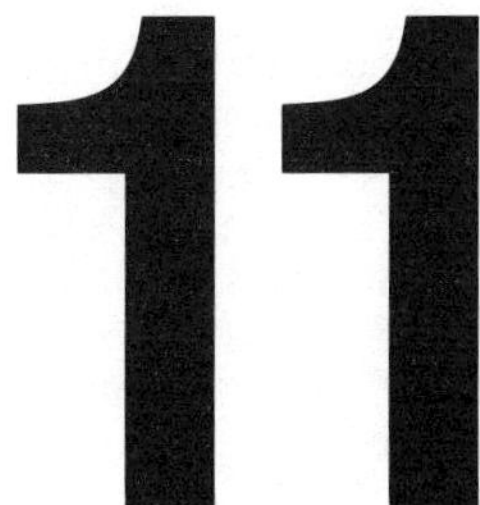

Dysrhythmias and Palpitations

Congenital heart disease is the most common underlying cardiac dysfunction in children. Dysrhythmias, although uncommon, may present as syncope, acute cardiac decompensation, palpitations, a feeling of "something different," or poor growth or feeding. Dysrhythmias are caused by abnormal impulse formation or conduction or by a combined mechanism.

Etiologic Considerations

1. Functional characteristics of the conduction system.
   a. Cardiac stimuli come from specialized neuromuscular tissues within the heart, consisting of the sinus (sinoatrial or SA) node, AV (atrioventricular) junction, bundle of His, right and left branches, and Purkinje fibers. The primary pacemaker is the sinus node and when this node is suppressed or fails to generate stimuli, another pacemaker becomes the rate setter. The stimuli become progressively slower as the site becomes more distal.
   b. Stimuli to the sinus node and AV junction are modified by sympathetic and vagal fibers. The sympathetic nervous system stimulates the heart while the vagal or parasympathetic system has a suppressive effect. Increased heart rate may result from increased sympathetic activity or decreased vagal tone while bradycardia is commonly due to increased vagal tone.
2. Disturbance of rhythm result when the rate is too fast *(tachycardia)* or too slow *(bradycardia)*. A number of factors contribute to the nature of the rhythm.
   a. Automatically occurs when myocardial tissue independently depolarizes, reaching threshold and then fires. It is increased by hypokalemia, hypercalcemia, catecholamines, drugs such as digitalis, and ischemia. Triggered automaticity occurs when the resting membrane potential is unstable following myocardial ischemia, fibrosis, or drug therapy (e.g., calcium, digitalis).
   b. Reentry dysrhythmias occur when a portion of the heart is depolarized while other areas are not. Reentry requires two pathways to be connected proximally and distally.
3. *Tachyrhythmias* result from increased sympathetic activity, decreased vagal tone, an ectopic pacemaker or a reentrant pathway that involves abnormal or accessory connections. Accessory pathways produce preexcitation syndromes such as Wolff-Parkinson-White (WPW), which predisposes to paroxysmal atrial tachycardia (PAT) or paroxysmal supraventricular tachycardia (PSVT).

   Patients with tachyrhythmias may present with palpitations, a minor sense of "uneasiness," or rapid progression of presenting signs and symptoms of congestive heart failure associated with shortness of breath, exercise intolerance, poor feeding, dizziness, and mental status changes. Patients with recurrent paroxysmal supraventricular tachycardia commonly recognize the presence of tachycardia and can often convert themselves with a variety of vagotonic maneuvers.
4. *Bradyrhythmias* are caused by slowing of the intrinsic pacemaker usually due to increased vagal tone or a conduction abnormality. Conduction blocks may be complete, in which circumstance a more distal, slower pacemaker controls the rate, or they may be incomplete, allowing only a few impulses to pass.

Bradycardia may cause syncope, lightheadedness, altered mental status, and ultimately cardiac standstill. Hypoxia is probably the most common cause of bradycardia.

Diagnostic Approach

Evaluation of the patient must focus on the following issues in determining both the etiology of the dysrhythmia and the stability of the patient:

- Does the patient have a dysrhythmia?
- Is the heart rate fast or slow?
- If the heart rate is fast, is the QRS wide (> 0.08 sec) or is it narrow?
- Is the patient unstable and therapy required?
- How soon is therapy required, if at all, and what is the most effective and safest therapy?

1. *History* should focus on presenting signs and symptoms, contributing factors, and current hemodynamic status.
   a. Presence of syncope, dizziness, lightheadedness, shortness of breath, exercise tolerance, chest pain, and mental status changes.
   b. Prior cardiac history including surgery, drugs, pacemaker, and so on.
   c. Ingestion of drugs, especially sympathomimetics such as cocaine, amphetamines, decongestants.
   d. Intercurrent infectious illness consistent with a viral process and concurrent myocarditis or pericarditis.
2. *Physical examination* should focus on the cardiac examination.
   a. Hemodynamic stability must be assessed by vital signs, including orthostatics.
   b. Rate, rhythm, murmurs, pulses, and chest require special focus.
   c. Exclude cardiac function by evaluating for ronchi, wheezing, jugular distension, edema, and hepatosplenomegaly.
3. *Diagnostic work-up*.
   a. Laboratory.
      (1) Complete blood count, electrolytes, calcium, and so on, as indicated.
      (2) Electrocardiogram (ECG) (Table 11-1).
         (a) Rate is age-dependent (newborn: 100–160, infant: 120–160, toddler: 80–150, child over 6 years: 60–120). Each small box on ECG paper is 0.04 seconds and time between vertical lines at top of strip is 3 seconds. Rate may be determined by multiplying the number of complexes between the veritcal lines by 20. *Determine if the rate is fast or slow.*
         (b) Axis is age specific, also reflecting hypertrophy or conduction defects.
         (c) Rhythm should be assessed for regularity and voltage. Voltage may be decreased in presence of myocarditis or effusion.
         (d) P wave implies atrial activity. It is seen best in leads II, III, and aVF. P wave may be enlarged or biphasic (V_1) implying atrial hypertropy. Normal width is 0.08–0.10 second.
         (e) PR interval represents a fixed relationship between the P wave and QRS interval and implies that the rhythm is supraventricular in origin. It is age-dependent and ranges from 0.10–0.20 second. Prolongation occurs with first degree-block, hyperkalemia, propranolol, verapamil, quinidine, and carditis. It is shortened in WPW.
         (f) QRS complex is normally less than 0.10 second. *Widened QRS complex generally implies a ventricular origin* or a conduction defect, severe hyperkalemia, or quinidine effect. Abnormal configuration demonstrates that the focus is ventricular in origin or that there is a conduction defect. High voltage occurs with hypertrophy or overload.
         (g) ST segment elevation occurs with transmural injury, pericarditis, or ventricular aneurysm. It may be depressed with subendocardial injury, digitalis, systolic overload, and strain.

(h) T wave peaks in hyperkalemia and is flat with hypokalemia. Conduction defect or ischemia may produce inversion.

(i) QT segment duration is rate dependent and is prolonged with quinidine, procainamide, tricyclic antidepressant overdose, hypokalemia, hypocalcemia, hypomagnesemia, and hypothermia.

(j) Other electrophysiologic studies may be indicated.

(i) Transtelephonic electrocardiography and Holter monitoring may be useful in defining dysrhythmias.

(ii) Supraventricular rhythms associated with syncope or frequent episodes of PSVT unresponsive to vagotonic maneuvers as well as ventricular rhythms associated with anatomical cardiac lesions may be studied. Sick sinus syndrome and AV conduction studies are also investigated as well.

b. Radiologic evaluation of the chest to investigate the heart for enlargement and the lungs for edema and fluid.

c. Therapeutic trials of vagotonic maneuvers including carotid message, Valsalva's maneuver, cold water applied to the face, coughing, and so on, result in increased vagal tone that should result in a transient slowing of the heart rate if the rhythm is supraventricular.

Alert: Description of any dysrhythmia must include whether the rate is fast or slow and if the QRS is wide or narrow. Hemodynamic stability determines the urgency of intervention.

Bibliography

Abramowicz M (ed): Drugs for cardiac arrhythmias. Med Lett Drug Ther 31:35, 1989.

Chameides JL: *Textbook of Pediatric Advanced Life Support*. Dallas: American Heart Association, 1988.

Harken AH, Honigman B, and VanWay CW: Cardiac dysrhythmias in the acute setting: recognition and treatment or anyone can treat dysrhythmias. J Emerg Med 5:129, 1987.

Moak J, et al: Newer antiarrhythmic drugs in children. Am Heart J 113:179, 1987.

Rosen M: Mechanisms of arrhythmias. Am J Cardiol 61:2A, 1988.

Table 11-1. Electrocardiographic Criteria

Age	Heart Rate (/min)	QRS Axis (degrees)	PR Interval (sec)	QRS Duration* (sec)
0–1 mo	100–180 (120)†	+75 to +180 (+120)	.08–.12 (.10)	.04–.08 (.06)
2–3 mo	110–180 (120)	+35 to +135 (+100)	.08–.12 (.10)	.04–.08 (.06)
4–12 mo	100–180 (150)	+30 to +135 (+60)	.09–.13 (.12)	.04–.08 (.06)
1–3 yr	100–180 (130)	0 to +110 (+60)	.10–.14 (.12)	.04–.08 (.06)
4–5 yr	60–150 (100)	0 to +110 (+60)	.11–.15 (.13)	.05–.09 (.07)
6–8 yr	60–130 (100)	−15 to +110 (+60)	.12–.16 (.14)	.05–.09 (.07)
9–11 yr	50–110 (80)	−15 to +110 (+60)	.12–.17 (.14)	.05–.09 (.07)
12–16 yr	50–100 (75)	−15 to +110 (+60)	.12–.17 (.15)	.05–.09 (.07)
>16 yr	50–90 (70)	−15 to +110 (+60)	.12–.20 (.15)	.05–.10 (.08)

QT Interval

Rate/min	R-R Interval (sec)	QT Interval (sec)
40	1.5	.38–.50 (.45)†
50	1.2	.36–.48 (.43)
60	1.0	.34–.46 (.41)
70	0.86	.32–.43 (.37)
80	0.75	.29–.40 (.35)
90	0.67	.27–.37 (.33)
100	0.60	.26–.35 (.30)
120	0.50	.24–.32 (.28)
150	0.40	.21–.28 (.25)
180	0.33	.19–.27 (.23)
200	0.30	.18–.25 (.22)

T-wave Orientation

Age	V1,V2	AVF	I,V5,V6
0–5 days	Variable	Upright	Upright
6 days–2 yr	Inverted	Upright	Upright
3 yr–adolescent	Inverted	Upright	Upright
Adult	Upright	Upright	Upright

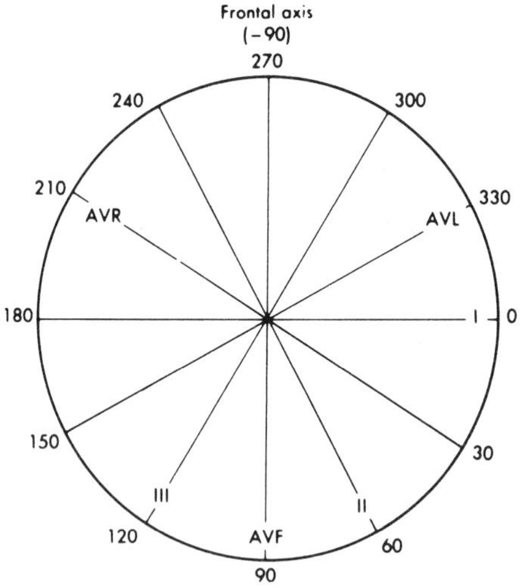

Frontal axis
(−90)
270
240
300
210
330
AVR
AVL
180
I
0
150
30
III
II
120
AVF
60
90

Adapted from Garson A, Jr, Gillette PC, and McNamara DG: A guide to cardiac dysrhythmias in children, New York, 1980, Grune & Stratton, Inc., and Guntheroth WGS: Pediatric electrocardiography, Philadelphia, 1965, WB Saunders Co. (Reproduced by permission from Barkin RM and Rosen P: *Emergency Pediatrics: A Guide to Ambulatory Care*, (3rd ed.). St. Louis: C. V. Mosby, 1990.)
*If QRS duration is normal, add R + R′ and compare total (R + R′) with standards; R/S undefined because S can be equal to 0.
†Minimum-maximum (mean).

Lead V1			Lead V6			
R-wave Amplitude (mm)	S-wave Amplitude (mm)	R/S Ratio	R-wave Amplitude (mm)	S-wave Amplitude (mm)	R/S Ratio	Age
4–25 (15)	0–20 (10)	0.5 to ∞ (1.5)	1–21 (6)	0–12 (4)	0.1 to ∞ (2)	0–1 mo
2–20 (11)	1–18 (7)	0.3 to 10.0 (1.5)	3–20 (10)	0–6 (2)	1.5 to ∞ (4)	2–3 mo
3–20 (10)	1–16 (8)	0.3 to 4.0 (1.2)	4–20 (13)	0–4 (2)	2.0 to ∞ (6)	4–12 mo
1–18 (9)	1–27 (13)	0.5 to 1.5 (0.8)	3–24 (12)	0–4 (2)	3.0 to ∞ (20)	1–3 yr
1–18 (7)	1–30 (14)	0.1 to 1.5 (0.7)	4–24 (13)	0–4 (1)	2.0 to ∞ (20)	4–5 yr
1–18 (7)	1–30 (14)	0.1 to 1.5 (0.7)	4–24 (13)	0–4 (1)	2.0 to ∞ (20)	6–8 yr
1–16 (6)	1–26 (16)	0.1 to 1.0 (0.5)	4–24 (14)	0–4 (1)	4.0 to ∞ (20)	9–11 yr
1–16 (5)	1–23 (14)	0 to 1.0 (0.3)	4–22 (14)	0–5 (1)	2.0 to ∞ (9)	12–16 yr
1–14 (3)	1–23 (10)	0 to 1.0 (0.3)	4–21 (10)	0–6 (1)	2.0 to ∞ (9)	>16 yr

Chamber enlargement ("hypertrophy")

Right ventricular

1. RV1 > 20 mm (>25 mm under 1 mo)
2. SV6 > 6 mm (>12 mm under 1 mo)
3. Abnormal R/S ratio (V1 > 2 after 6 mo)
4. Upright TV3R, RV1 after 5 days
5. QR pattern in V3R, V1

Left ventricular

1. RV6 > 25 mm (>21 mm under 1 yr)
2. SV1 > 30 mm (>20 mm under 1 yr)
3. RV6 + SV1 > 60 mm (Use V5 if RV5 > RV6)
4. Abnormal R/S ratio
5. SV1 > 2 × RV5

Combined

1. RVH and SV1 or RV6 exceed mean for age
2. LVH and RV1 or SV6 exceed mean for age

Right atrial

1. Peak P valve > 3 mm (<6 mo), >2.5 mm (≥6 mo)

Left atrial

1. PII > 0.09 sec
2. PV1 late negative deflection > 0.04 sec and > 1 mm

Maximal PR Interval (sec)

Rate/min	<1 mo	1 mo–1 yr	1–3 yr	3–8 yr	8–12 yr	Adult
<60					0.18	0.21
60–80				0.17	0.17	0.21
80–100	0.12			0.16	0.16	0.20
100–120	0.12		0.16	0.16	0.15	0.19
120–140	0.11	0.14	0.14	0.15	0.15	0.18
140–160	0.11	0.13	0.14	0.14		0.17
>160	0.11	0.11				

12 Hypertension

Children with hypertension have systolic or diastolic blood pressures above the 95 percentile for age and sex (Table 12-1). The assessment of blood pressure requires the use of an appropriately sized cuff, usually covering about two-thirds of the child's upper arm. The inflatable bladder should encircle the arm without overlapping. Too narrow a cuff will give a false elevation of blood pressure, while too wide a cuff may give a low reading. Cuffs are available for premature infants (4 cm wide), larger babies (5 and 7 cm wide), and children (9, 13, and 15.5 cm). In older children, the auscultatory method is used while palpation, flush, or Doppler approaches are useful in infants. When the measurement is elevated in one arm, blood pressure should be assessed in the other arm as well as the lower extremities.

Etiologic Considerations

Hypertension may be classified as primary or secondary. Primary, or *essential*, hypertension is rare but may occur in older children, while secondary hypertension is due to a variety of conditions. Elevated blood pressure in children under 12 years is usually associated with anatomic pathology (Table 12-2).

1. *Neonates*: coarctation of the aorta, renovascular disease, and intracranial hemorrhage.
2. Up to 2 years of age: renovascular disease, intrinsic renal disease (cystic, hydronephrosis, pyelonephritis and Wilm's tumor), coarctation of the aorta, and neuroblastoma.
3. From 2–8 years of age: renovascular or intrinsic renal disease (cystic, pyelonephritis).
4. Over 8 years of age: renovascular disease, intrinsic renal disease (cystic, pyelonephritis, glomerulonephritis, and collagen), essential hypertension.

Most patients with mild hypertension are asymptomatic, but as pressure increases a variety of central nervous and cardiovascular signs and symptoms may develop.

1. Hypertensive encephalopathy including headache, confusion, vomiting, and anorexia with mental status deterioration. Visual blurring with transient blindness may accompany retinal hemorrhages, exudates, and papilledema.
2. Intracerebral or subarachnoid hemorrhage.
3. Cardiac decompensation. Low blood pressure may be due to a variety of conditions causing hypovolemic, cardiogenic, or distributive shock (Chap. 3).

Diagnostic Approach

1. *History* should focus on the presentation, potential causes, and underlying conditions.
   a. Central nervous system findings including headache, changing mental status, or visual disturbances.
   b. Cardiac decompensation manifested by shortness of breath, chest pain, weakness, or dizziness.
   c. Evidence of renal or vascular disease.

Table 12-1. Hypertension by Age (95 percentile)

Age	Systolic Pressure	Diastolic Pressure
Premature	80 mm Hg	45 mm Hg
Term infant	90 mm Hg	60 mm Hg
0–6 months	110 mm Hg	60 mm Hg
3 yr	112 mm Hg	80 mm Hg
5 yr	115 mm Hg	84 mm Hg
10 yr	130 mm Hg	92 mm Hg
15 yr	140 mm Hg	95 mm Hg

Table 12-2. Common Causes of Secondary Hypertension

Renal parenchymal disease
- Glomerulonephritis
- Pyelonephritis
- Henoch-Schonlein purpura (HSP)
- Hemolytic uremic syndrome (HUS)
- Polycystic kidney disease
- Dysplastic kidney
- Obstructive uropathy
- Autoimmune disease

Renal vascular disease
- Arterial anomalies or thrombosis
- Venous anomalies or thrombosis

Vascular disease
- Coarctation of the aorta
- Dissection of leaking aortic aneurysm
- Renal artery stenosis
- Vasculitis
- Aortic or mitral insufficiency

Neurologic disease
- Encephalitis
- Brain tumor

Endocrine disease
- Pheochromocytoma
- Steroid therapy, oral contraceptives
- Toxemia of pregnancy
- Hyperthyroidism

Intoxication
- Sympathomimetics: amphetamines, hallucinogens (LSD)
- Heavy metal: lead, mercury
- MAO inhibitor accompanied by use of alcohol or ripened cheese (e.g., Brie, cheddar) containing tyramine (produces catecholamine release)

Anxiety, usually producing labile changes

2. *Physical examination* must include correct measurement of the blood pressure and assessment of potential complications. Particular attention must be paid to rapidity of onset and rise of blood pressure and evidence of systemic compromise resulting from the increased pressure.
   a. Measurement of blood pressure with orthostatic assessment on several occasions. Use correct cuff size and measurement of multiple extremities.
   b. Central nervous system, cardiac, and peripheral vascular examination.
   c. Other sequelae or indications of systemic disease.
3. *Diagnostic approach.*
   a. Laboratory.
      (1) Urinalysis and urine culture. Twenty-four-hour urine for protein and creatinine clearance.

Calculation of Creatinine Clearance

Creatinine clearance (ml/min/1.73 m^2) $= \frac{UV}{P} \times \frac{1.73}{SA}$

U = urinary concentration of creatinine (mg/dl)
V = volume of urine divided by the number of minutes in collection period (24 hr = 1440 min) (ml/min)
P = plasma concentration of creatinine (mg/dl)
SA = surface area (m^2)

Normal newborn and premature: 40–65 ml/min/1.73 m^2
Normal child: 109 (female) or 124 (male) ml/min/1.73 m^2
Adult: 95 (female) or 105 (male) ml/min/1.73 m^2

      (2) Chemistry: BUN and creatinine (see above). Consider electrolytes, calcium, and phosphorus.
      (3) ECG.
      (4) Other studies as indicated for specific contributing causes.
   b. Radiologic studies should include a chest x-ray.

Alert: Rapid onset or progression of hypertension may result in cardiac and central nervous system decompensation requiring emergent evaluation and intervention.

Bibliography

Abramowicz M (ed): Drugs for hypertensive emergencies. Med Lett Drug Ther 31:25, 1989.

Buchi KF and Siegler RL: Hypertension in the first month of life. J Hypertens 4:525, 1986.

Farine M and Arbus GS: Management of hypertensive emergencies in children. Pediatr Emerg Care 5:51, 1989.

Report on the Second Task Force on blood pressure control in children – 1987. Task force on blood pressure control in children. National Heart, Lung and Blood Institute. Bethesda, MD, Pediatrics 79:1, 1987.

V Dermatologic Problems

13 Rash

Rashes represent an acute skin eruption, commonly reflecting an infectious etiology in children. Categorization of the rash after careful physical examination and description is necessary to identify the underlying disease. Describing the lesion is essential (Tables 13-1 and 13-2).

Etiologic Considerations

The majority of rashes in children are acute, representing a dermatologic presentation of an underlying infectious disease (Table 13-3).

Differential entities must be evaluated in a systematic manner to assure appropriate evaluation. In assessing a specific rash, first determine if it is *fluid-filled* or *solid* and if solid, define if it is *red* or *nonred* and *scaling* or *nonscaling*.

Diagnostic Approach

1. *History* should focus on the rash and associated signs and symptoms.
   a. Pattern of rash with respect to onset, progression, and distribution.
   b. Associated pruritus, scaling, bruising, and pain, often worsening with sun exposure.
   c. Accompanying signs and symptoms.
2. *Physical examination*.
   a. Assess stability of patient and define findings.
   b. Describe appearance, number, pattern, distribution, size, spread, and nature of rash.
3. *Diagnostic work-up* is rarely required except to exclude specific diagnostic entities. Gram's stain or culture may be helpful.

   Therapeutic trial is often useful in defining both the etiologic process as well as therapeutic options. Often topical treatment quickly results in resolution and rapid identification of many problems, usually of a nonsystemic nature.

Alert: Patients with conditions requiring attention include those with lesions that are purple (purpura), do not blanch (petechiae), are burnlike (scaled skin), are blue or tender to the touch (cellulitis), have red streaking (lymphangitis), or are pustular.

Bibliography

American Academy of Pediatrics: *Report of the Committee on Infectious Diseases*, 21st ed. Elk Grove Village: American Academy of Pediatrics, 1988.

Weston WL: *Practical Pediatric Dermatology* (2d ed.). Boston: Little, Brown, 1985.

Table 13-1. Rash: Dermatologic Category

Appearance	Etiologic Considerations
Solid, Nonred	
Skin-colored	*Keratotic*, rough-surfaced: wart, callus, corn *Nonkeratotic*, smooth-surfaced: wart, mulloscum contagiosum, nevi
Brown	Café-au-lait patch, nevi, freckle, hypopigmentation secondary to systemic disease, medication, or post-inflammatory condition
Yellow	Jaundice, nevi sebaceous
White	Pityriasis alba, post-inflammatory hypopigmentation
Solid, Red, Nonscaling	
Inflammatory papule/nodule	*Papule/maculopapule*: viral exanthem (measles, rubella, roseola, enterovirus), erythema multiforme, scarlatina, drug reaction (Table 13-3) *Nodule*: furuncle, erythema nodosum
Vascular, flat	*Nonpurpuric*, erythema: toxic (viral, medication), urticaria (infection, medication), erythema multiforme, cellulitis (erysipelas) *Purpuric/petechiae*: viral (enterovirus), rubeola (atypical), sepsis *(N. meningococcus, H. influenzae)*, ecchymosis, vasculitis (Henoch-Schonlein purpura), cough
Solid, Red, Scaling	
Papulosquamous	Pityriasis rosea, tinea corporis
Eczematous	Atopic, dermatitis (seborrhea, diaper, contact), tinea cruris or capitus, impetigo, candidiasis
Blister, Fluid Filled	
Vesicle (Table 13-4)	Herpes simplex/zoster, chickenpox, scabies
Bullae	Bullous impetigo, erythema multiforme, burn
Pustule	Acne, folliculitis, candidiasis, bacteremia

Table 13-2. Dermatologic Lesions

Macule:	color change that is flat and not palpable. If greater than 1 cm, it is called a **Patch**.
Papule:	small (< 1 cm), firm, elevated lesion with distinct borders.
Vesicle:	papule filled with clear fluid. If greater than 1 cm, it is a **bullae**.
Pustule:	papule filled with exudate.
Nodule:	raised, palpable lesion with indistinct border.
Papulosquamous:	red or violaceous lesion that may progress to papules and develop scales; no epithelial disruption.
Eczematous:	epithelial disruption.

Table 13-3. Maculopapular Exanthem

	Incubation	Prodrome	Exanthem	Other Findings
Measles (Rubeola)	10–14 days	Fever, cough, conjunctivitis, coryza; toxic	Reddish-brown; begins on face and becomes confluent	Koplik's spots; pneumonia, encephalitis, otitis media
Rubella (3-day measles)	14–21 days	Minimal; lymphadenopathy	Pink, discrete, begins on face	Arthritis, encephalitis
Roseola (exanthema subitum)	10–14 days	3–4 days high fever, preceding rash	Rose, discrete; appears after defervescence	Febrile seizure
Fifth disease (erythema infectiosum)	7–14 days	None	Red-flushed cheeks; eruption extremity may reoccur	Arthritis
Enterovirus	Variable	Fever, malaise, sore throat	Discrete, generalized; hand-foot-mouth	Aseptic meningitis, myocarditis
Scarlatina (see also p. 276)	2–4 days	Fever, vomiting, sore throat	Erythematous, punctate, sandpaper; flexor surface; skin folds	Group A streptococcus, staphylococcus; rheumatic fever, acute glomerulonephritis

Table 13-4. Vesicular Exanthems

	Incubation	Exanthem	Other Findings
Varicella (chickenpox) (see also p. 268)	14–21 days	Erythematous macule progressing to papule and vesicle; pruritic; central, distal sparing	Mucosal ulcers, dehydration; pneumonia, secondary bacterial infection; encephalitis; Reye's
Herpes zoster (shingles)	Variable	Erythema followed by papules and vesicles in 12–24 hours, pustule in 72 hours and crusts in 10–12 days; follows dermatome	Ophthalmic neuralgia, corneal dendrite; postherpetic neuralgia
Herpes simplex	Variable	Erythema progressing to vesicle	Gingivostomatitis, vulvovaginitis, keratoconjunctivitis; corneal ulcer, encephalitis, neonatal viremia

VI

Ear, Nose, and Throat Problems

14 Ear Pain

Earache or otalgia is common in children, often associated with middle ear infection. It is essential to consider the breadth of differential considerations before initiating specific therapy (Table 14-1). Ear pain may be caused by ear pathology or by referral from another facial area. Conditions having associated ear pain may include upper respiratory infections, thyroiditis, dental pathology, and difficulty in swallowing due to esophageal or gastric disease. (See also p. 257.)

Diagnostic Considerations

Hearing loss may often go unnoticed until language impairment becomes obvious. Types of hearing loss assist in differentiating causes and therapeutic approaches:

1. Conductive due to impairment in the external auditory canal, eardrum, ossicular chain, middle ear cavity, the oval window, or the round window. Correction may be achieved medically or surgically.
2. Sensorineural hearing loss may occur from damage to the cochlear part of the auditory system (sensory) or the auditory nerve (neural). The loss is irreversible.
3. Functional hearing loss has no organic basis.
4. Central auditory dysfunction is secondary to central nervous system.

Diagnostic Approach

1. *History* should focus on the nature of the pain, its location, and previous episodes.
   a. Onset, severity, radiation and progression of pain. Factors that reduce or worsen discomfort. Pain over mastoid or with movement of pinna.
   b. Associated audiologic and respiratory tract involvement and systemic findings including fever, impaired mental status, and changed behavior.
   c. Children that have had their first episode of otitis media in the first year of life are *prone* to have additional cases in subsequent years.
2. *Physical examination.*
   a. Examine the external ear and ear canal and inspect the middle ear visually and with otoscope.
      (1) External canal and mastoid. Pain with movement of pinna.
      (2) Tympanic membrane color, mobility, landmarks. Pneumatic otoscopy is essential.
   b. Potential secondary conditions should be excluded. A large number of cases of meningitis are associated with otitis media and a careful evaluation of neurologic status and alertness is essential.
   c. Associated fever, respiratory tract findings.
3. *Diagnostic work-up* of any extent is only indicated to evaluate the patient for specific pathology. Commonly, no laboratory data is required but specific conditions may necessitate more in-depth studies. Those with significant or recurrent ear problems should have their hearing assessed.

Table 14-1. Ear Pain: Etiologic Considerations

Condition	Diagnostic Findings	Comments
Infection		
Otitis media acute (AOM)	Tympanic membrane is red, immobile; fever, irritability; variable hearing loss; perforation rare; conductive hearing loss common	Must differentiate from systemic infection
Otitis media external	Severe pain, particularly upon movement of tragus; systemic signs uncommon	Foreign body may be contributory
Bullous myringitis	Acute severe pain accompanied by bullae on tympanic membrane	Mycoplasma and other pathogens
Mastoiditis	Pain, edema, tenderness over mastoid area. Postauricular swelling	Uncommon complication of otitis media
Peritonsillar abscess (Chap. 17)	Toxic; severe sore throat, progressive trismus, drooling, unilateral tonsillar displacement	Aspiration for diagnosis and management
Sinusitis	Rhinorrhea, cough worse at night, local tenderness	Clinical diagnosis; x-ray confirmation
Parotitis	Localized swelling, tenderness over parotid	Mumps is most common
Lymphadenitis (Chap. 15)	Swelling, tenderness, and warmth	Usually cervical or post-auricular
Trauma		
Foreign body	History with evidence of foreign body or unilateral drainage	Often accompanied by external otitis media
Barotrauma	Acute onset of pain with change in air pressure	Diving or flying with altitude change
Penetrating trauma	Acute onset of pain; perforation often present	ENT evaluation
Impacted third molar	Abnormal position or infection (caries)	Dental evaluation
Temporomandibular joint dysfunction (Chap. 34)	Recurrent ear and facial pain; headache	Evaluate stress
Allergic		
Otitis media serous	Intermittent sharp or dull pain; hearing deficit	Check hearing

Alert: Meningitis may accompany an ear infection and must be excluded on the basis of history and physical examination. If uncertainty remains, a lumbar puncture is indicated.

Bibliography

Kramer H and Kramer AM: The phantom earache: temporomandibular joint dysfunction in children. Am J Dis Child 139:943, 1985.

Mandel EM, Rockette HE, and Bluestone CD: Efficacy of amoxicillin with and without decongestant-antihistamine for otitis media with effusion in children: results of a double blind, randomized trial. N Engl J Med 316:432, 1987.

Paradise J: Otitis media in infants and children. Pediatrics 65:917, 1980.

Teele D, Klein J, and Rosner B: Epidemiology of otitis media in children. Ann Otol Rhinol Laryngol 89:S5, 1980.

15 Lymphadenopathy and Neck Swelling

Lymph nodes are variably palpable in normal infants and children in the cervical, axillary, inguinal, and occipital regions. Thirty four percent of neonates (< 4 weeks) have palpable nodes in one or more sites while head and neck nodes are palpable in 45% of normal children.

Etiologic Considerations

The presence of localized adenopathy indicates that there is drainage to an infected area. If no infection exists, other etiologies must be considered, requiring an extensive evaluation. Systemic disease may initially present with localized lymphadenopathy, and generalized lymphadenopathy is also usually indicative of a systemic disease.

Diagnostic Approach

In addition to the routine evaluation, an empiric course of antibiotics for patients with localized lymphadenopathy may be useful while watching the course of the lymphadenopathy and associated signs and symptoms carefully (Table 15-1).

1. *History* often uncovers symptoms associated with the mass effect of the node enlargement and involvement of underlying structures.
   a. Fever and systemic toxicity.
   b. Onset, duration, and progression of lymphadenopathy.
   c. Evidence of complications including dysphagia, difficulty breathing (usually obstructive if cervical lymphadenopathy), stridor, cyanosis, cough, respiratory distress, and edema of face.
   d. Abdominal pain associated with mesenteric and retroperitoneal lymphadenopathy and, rarely, iliac adenitis.
   e. Other associated symptoms. (Exclude mumps, see page 264.)

2. *Physical examination* should define the location and nature of the lymph node enlargement.
   a. Location of the lymphadenopathy and assessment for size, tenderness, overlying erythema, and fluctuance. Differential considerations of cervical lymphadenopathy may include parotitis, which may anatomically be difficult to distinguish, congenital bronchial cleft or thyroglossal duct cyst, hemangioma, or cystic hygroma.
   b. Stiffness of the neck accompanying cervical lymphadenopathy. Other considerations in the child with a stiff neck must include meningitis, trauma with muscle spasm or hematoma, torticollis, spinal osteomyelitis, and peritonsillar and retropharyngeal abscess.
   c. Evidence of systemic disease.

3. *Diagnostic work-up*
   a. Laboratory
      (1) Complete blood count.
      (2) Monospot and other serologies for specific etiologies.

Table 15-1. Lymphadenopathy: Etiologic Considerations

Condition	Diagnostic Findings	Comments
Infection		
Bacterial	Rapid onset with warmth, erythema, tenderness	Usually obvious source of infection and localized enlargement (Staphylococcus, group A streptococcus, tularemia, plague, diphtheria)
Viral	Insidious onset with minimal tenderness	Rubella (post-auricular, post-cervical, occipital); Mononucleosis (post-cervical); Roseola
Cat scratch fever	Localized, depending upon site of scratch. Node nontender, discrete, moveable; variable systemic findings	May persist for 1–4 weeks
Tuberculosis	Systemic illness; generalized (hematogenous) or localized (mediastinal, cervical) nodes	Exposure, skin test; atypical is usually cervical
Mucocutaneous lymph node syndrome (Kawasaki syndrome)	Fever, conjunctival injection, mouth fissuring, erythema, edema, erythematous rash, coronary artery disease	Under 5 years; acute to subacute to convalescent phase; cardiac sequelae
Other Protozoa (toxoplasmosis, trypanosomiasis) Fungal (histoplasmosis, dermatophytosis) Spirochete (syphilis, leptospirosis)	Variable presentation	
Neoplasm		
Primary (Hodgkin) Secondary Leukemia Histiocytoses Neuroblastoma Thyroid	Variable presentation; often supraclavicular (spread via thoracic duct) or unusual locations	
Miscellaneous		
Autoimmune	Variable systemic presentation	
Hypersensitivity Serum sickness Drug reaction	Known exposure to parenteral agent; fever, systemic illness	
Storage disease Niemann-Pick		
AIDS		

(3) Streptozyme and throat culture for group A streptococcus (cervical lymphadenopathy).
(4) Intermediate-strength purified protein derivative (PPD) test (usually < 10 mm with atypical disease but may be negative).
(5) Aspiration or biopsy of the enlarged node for histologic and microbiologic assessment.
(6) Other studies may include bone marrow examination, immunologic evaluation, and other tissue inspection.

b. Radiologic evaluation by chest x-ray, CT scan of abdomen and chest, and so on, to look for specific systemic disease.

Alert: Infection is commonly the underlying cause of lymphadenopathy; in the face of enlargement that is unresponsive to antibiotics, it is essential to monitor closely while looking for underlying disease.

Bibliography

American Academy of Pediatrics: *Report of the Committee on Infectious Diseases*, 21st ed. Elk Grove: American Academy of Pediatrics, 1988.

Bamji M, Stone RK, Kaul A, et al.: Palpable lymph nodes in healthy newborns and infants. Pediatrics 78:573, 1986.

English CK, West DT, Margileth AM, et al.: Cat-scratch disease. JAMA 259:1347, 1988.

16 Nasal Discharge and Epistaxis

Nasal discharge is commonly mucopurulent when infectious in origin, while trauma often produces bleeding or epistaxis. (See also p. 243.)

Etiologic Considerations

1. *Nasal discharge* may result from a variety of infectious origins or, less commonly, a foreign body.
   a. Rhinitis.
      Viral: rhinovirus, influenza, respiratory syncytial virus (RSV), parainfluenza.
      Bacterial: *C. diphtheriae, H. influenzae, S. pneumoniae.*
   b. Sinusitis presents with rhinorrhea, purulent discharge, cough that is worse at night, sinus pain, and headache. Bacterial: *H. influenzae* (19–32%), *S. pneumoniae* (9–28%), group A streptococcus (17–27%), *S. aureus* (6–21%).
   c. Trauma: foreign body.
2. *Nasal bleeding* producing epistaxis originates in the anterior portion of the nasal septum (Kiesselbach's area) in 90% of patients. Differential conditions producing bleeding include:
   a. Trauma: nose picking, foreign body, blunt trauma, repeated blowing associated with rhinitis.
   b. Allergic rhinitis or polyp.
   c. Bleeding dyscrasia: congenital abnormality, aspirin ingestion, anticoagulant, neoplasm.
   d. Vascular: telangiectasia, hemangioma.

Diagnostic Approach

1. *History* should determine if the infection is the likely underlying illness.
   a. Respiratory tract infections, including rhinorrhea, fever, posterior nasal drip, cough, and headache. Repetitive response to inhalation exposure and consistent allergic reaction.
   b. History of trauma or foreign body. Foreign body is often associated with unilateral, odorific discharge.
   c. Bleeding diathesis or drug ingestion.
2. *Physical examination* should include a full evaluation of the nose after hemodynamic stability has been ensured. Also evaluate for sinus tenderness and upper respiratory tract infection.
3. *Laboratory* evaluation is usually limited but may include specific tests to exclude specific conditions.
   a. Microbiologic examination of discharge for PMN's or eosinophils (allergy).
   b. Bleeding screen (PT, PTT, platelets, bleeding time) if there is associated excessive bleeding (Chap. 30).
   c. Sinus radiographs in older children as indicated.

Alert: Discharge is commonly due to a URI; possibility of a foreign body must be excluded.

Bibliography

Chanin A: Prevention of recurrent nosebleeds in children. Clin Pediatr (Phila) 11:684, 1972.

Juselius H: Epistaxis: a clinical study of 1734 patients. J Laryngol Otol 88:317, 1974.

17 Pharyngitis or Sore Throat

Most children with a sore throat or painful sensation of the pharynx and surrounding tissues have an accompanying pharyngitis of a self-limited nature, but more significant conditions may be underlying (Table 17-1). (See also p. 277.)

Etiologic Considerations

The dominant cause of sore throat in children is infection. The etiologic agent is differentiated through the child's history in combination with laboratory support. Less common entities should be excluded. *Exudative pharyngitis* accompanies group A streptococci, EB virus (infectious mononucleosis), *Corynebacterium diphtheriae*, and adenovirus. Exudate is commonly associated with a virus in children younger than 3 years and by group A streptococcus in those older than 6. *Soft-palatal petechiae* are found with group A streptococcal and EB virus infections; *vesicles* or *ulcers* on the posterior tonsillar pillars with enterovirus infection; and *ulcers* on the anterior palate with herpes infections.

Diagnostic Approach

1. *Historically*, the focus is necessarily on the nature of the sore throat and associated findings.
   a. Onset, progression, and severity of sore throat.
   b. Associated fever, toxicity, respiratory findings, difficulty swallowing or breathing, lymphadenopathy, ear or dental pain, or systemic findings. Cough is rarely found in children with group A streptococcal infections.
   c. Exposure to infection at home, school, day care, or work.
   d. Prior history of similar infections. History of recurrent sore throats that are culture proven (usually unreliable unless there is good documentation). Previous immunologic studies to exclude carrier state.
2. *Physical examination* is primarily of the throat and neck regions.
   a. Pharyngeal examination must be thorough. Evaluate pharynx for erythema, petechiae, fluctuance; tonsils for erythema, fluctuance, enlargement; uvula for deviation; teeth for caries and abscess.
   b. Complete evaluation for other systemic findings.
3. *Diagnostic work-up*.
   a. Laboratory assessment may include:
      (1) Throat culture for group A streptococcus.
         (a) Initially, a rapid simple diagnostic test is available for early diagnosis. However, in view of the high false negative rate, it is essential to confirm negative tests with a routine culture.
         (b) Positive cultures with a low colony count may be indicative of the carrier state. To investigate this possibility, a Streptozyme must be ordered. Low titers are consistent with a chronic carrier state.
         (c) Infants should have their noses rather than throats cultured.

Table 17-1. Pharyngitis: Etiologic Considerations

Condition	Diagnostic findings	Comments
Infection		
Pharyngitis (Chap. 17)		
Viral	Sore throat, cough, rhinitis, conjunctivitis (adenovirus), congestion, variably tender adenitis; herpangina (enterovirus: fever, dysphagia, vesicle soft palate); normal WBC, negative throat culture	Influenzae, herpes simplex, EB virus (mononucleosis often with exudate), adenovirus, enterovirus
Bacterial	Sore throat; variable toxicity, fever, exudate, headache, abdominal pain, systemic findings; listless; scarlatinaform rash; elevated WBC, positive throat culture	Group A streptococcus; other: *N. gonorrhea* or *meningitidis, C. diphtheria, Mycoplasma pneumoniae, Chlamydia*
Epiglottitis (Chap. 46)	Acute onset of "worst" sore throat, difficulty breathing; toxic, drooling, stridor; epiglottis enlarged; elevated WBC	*H. influenzae*; must differentiate from croup
Herpetic stomatitis	Rapid onset sore throat, usually localized to anterior buccal mucosa; ulcers, erosions; culture positive	Differentiate from aphthous stomatitis (canker sores)
Peritonsillar abscess	Sore throat with bulging posterior soft palate; deviation uvula to contralateral side; fluctuance	May follow pharyngitis; often group A streptococcus; adolescents
Retropharyngeal abscess	Sore throat, toxicity, difficult swallowing, variable respiratory distress; soft tissue x-ray: fullness of retropharyngeal tissue	Infrequent; usually children < 4 yr
Cervical lymphadenitis (Chap. 15)	Fever, enlarged, variably tender nodes, variable systemic findings	Commonly viral or group A streptococcus; referred pain
Otitis media (Chap. 14)	Ear pain; variable fever, systemic findings	Referred pain
Dental abscess	Localized findings	Referred pain
Psychiatric		
Globus hystericus	Difficulty swallowing	
Trauma		
Foreign body	Foreign body such as fishbone may be lodged in pharynx; x-ray	

(2) Rarely, other organisms should be sought.
(3) WBC may be useful in defining group A streptococcal infection.

b. Radiograph of the neck, if applicable.

c. Therapeutic trial of penicillin therapy may be considered. Children with group A streptococcal infections clinically respond rapidly. Note: Patients may return to work or school 24 hours after beginning therapy.

Alert: The severity of signs and symptoms is helpful in delineating the nature of the evaluation.

Bibliography

Bass JW: Treatment of streptococcal pharyngitis revisited. JAMA 256:740, 1986.

Berkowitz CD, Anthony BF, Kaplan EL, et al.: Cooperative study of latex agglutination to identify group A streptococcal antigen on throat swabs in patients with acute pharyngitis. J Pediatr 107:89, 1985.

Dillon H: Streptococcal pharyngitis in the 1980's. Pediatr Infect Dis J 6:123, 1987.

Putto A: Febrile exudative tonsillitis: viral or streptococcal. Pediatrics 80:6, 1987.

VII

Eye Problems

18 Impaired Vision

A disturbance in vision must be assessed with respect to the age-appropriate acuity normal. A 5-year-old normally has a visual acuity of 20/30, a 4-year-old typically has 20/40, while a 3-year-old can have normal vision with an acuity of 20/50.

Etiologic Considerations

A variety of conditions lead to disturbance of vision either on an acute or prolonged basis. *Acute* impairment is most commonly due to trauma (chemical burns, hyphema, rupture of globe, periorbital injury, or cortical blindness) or conjunctivitis. Alkali burns and central retinal artery occlusion must be treated *emergently* (Table 18-1).

Diagnostic Approach

1. *Historical* data can be useful with respect to etiology.
   a. Rapidity of onset and progression.
   b. Associated injury, infection, systemic disease, prior problems.
2. *Physical examination* must include a complete eye examination.
   a. Visual acuity using the picture card, "E," or Snellen chart. A difference of more than two lines between the eyes is probably more significant than the absolute acuity suggestive of refractive error, amblyopia, or trauma.
   b. External examination focusing on orbital bones, infraorbital nerve, lids, globe, cornea, anterior chamber, pupil (size, reactivity, regularity) and ocular mobility.
   c. Fundoscopic examination.
   d. Fluorescein staining.
3. *Diagnostic work-up* is rarely required beyond a careful examination. If there is a question of blowout bone fracture or radioopaque foreign body, an x-ray film may be appropriate.
   Alert: Acute onset of impaired visual acuity usually necessitates ophthalmologic evaluation.

Bibliography

Grin TR, Nelson LB, Jeffers JF: Eye injuries in childhood. Pediatrics 80:13, 1987.

Table 18-1. Impaired Vision: Etiologic Considerations

Condition	Diagnostic Findings	Comments
Infection		
Conjunctivitis (Chap. 19)	Conjunctival erythema, variable vision and cornea	Bacterial, viral, *Chlamydia*
Cellulitis	Erythema, warmth, swelling of lip; minimal conjunctivitis	*H. influenzae, S. aureus, S. pneumoniae*
Trauma		
Eyelid hematoma, edema, laceration	Preceding blunt or penetrating trauma	
Chemical, thermal, ultraviolet burn	Fluorescein staining; watery discharge; foreign body pain	Alkali burn is medical emergency
Corneal abrasion	Fluorescein staining; foreign body sensation	
Hyphema	Blood in anterior chamber	Blunt trauma
Cataract/ lens dislocation	Cloudy or displaced lens	Blunt trauma
Head trauma (Chap. 47)	Transient cortical blindness resolving over time	Blunt head trauma
Other		
Refractive error	Careful testing and correction	Myopia, hyperopia, astigmatism
Strabismus	Abnormal eye movement	Inequality of musculature
Amblyopia	Unequal visual acuity	Due to strabismus, unequal refraction, unilateral disease
Glaucoma	Increased intraocular pressure	
Retinal vein/ artery occlusion	Vein: painless loss of vision; hemorrhages of fundus, blurred disc Artery: sudden, painless loss of vision; field loss; cherry-red spot of fovea, pale disc	Thrombi (endocardial, trauma, cystic fibrosis, SLE, sickle cell disease); artery occlusion-emergency
Retinal detachment	Loss of vision	Spontaneous, trauma
Neuritis	Associated findings	
Toxin	Variable pattern, associated signs and symptoms	Methanol, halogenated hydrocarbon, quinine, salicylate
Migraine (Chap. 34)	Headache, bilateral transient field loss, nausea; scotomata	

19 Red Eyes

Eye problems commonly present with vascular dilation, pain, and reflex tear secretion. A variety of etiologies are causative (Table 19-1). (See also p. 258.)

Diagnostic Approach

1. The *history* must focus on potential etiologic conditions.
   - **a.** Onset, progression, and nature of redness.
   - **b.** Presence of eye pain, trauma, radiation, drug, chemical exposure.
   - **c.** Preceding trauma.
   - **d.** Systemic signs and symptoms.
2. *Physical examination* must define eye pathology.
   - **a.** Examination of external and internal eye including fundus and tonometry.
   - **b.** Visual acuity.
   - **c.** Slit lamp exam may be required.
   - **d.** Fluorescein examination to exclude foreign body and corneal abrasion.
3. *Diagnostic work-up* is usually not necessary unless there are specific concerns.
   - **a.** Cultures, fluorescent antibody, or Gram's stain of discharge may be appropriate for infection in the newborn, particularly if purulent (*N. gonorrhoeae*) or associated with pneumonia (*Chlamydia trachomatis*).
   - **b.** Radiograph for foreign body if metallic body suspected.

   Alert: Eye pain, decreased visual acuity, or persistence of signs and symptoms should indicate a reasonable commitment.

Bibliography

Gigliotti F, Williams WT, Hayden FG, et al.: Etiology of acute conjunctivitis in children. Pediatrics 98:531, 1981.

Heggie AD, Jaffe AC, Stuart LA, et al.: Topical sulfacetamide vs. oral erythromycin for neonatal chlamydial conjunctivitis. Am J Dis Child 139:564, 1985.

Table 19-1. Red Eye: Etiologic Considerations

Condition	History	Vision	Discharge	Cornea	Conjunctiva	Other
Bacterial *S. pneumoniae* *S. haemophilus*	Bilateral, exposure	Normal	Purulent, PMNs	Normal	Injected	Painless
Viral Adenovirus	Exposure, systemic symptoms	Down	Mucoid, monos	Punctuate keratopathy	Injected	FBS, incubation 5–14 days
Herpes simplex	Unilateral	Variable	Mucoid, mono	Dendrite	Injected	FBS, photophobia
Chlamydia	Recurrent newborn	Normal	Inclusion body	Normal	Injected	Pneumonia
Trauma						
Foreign body/ Corneal abrasion	Trauma	Variable	None	Stain*	Injected	FBS
Radiation burn	Sun lamp, snow	Down	Watery	Stain*	Injected	FBS, photophobia
Chemical burn	Alkali worse than acid	Down	Watery	Hazy to opacified	Normal to blanched	FBS, photophobia
Other						
Allergy	Exposure	Normal	Watery	Normal	Injected	Seasonal
Glaucoma	Premature	Down	Watery	Cloudy	Injected	High pressure Mid size pupil
Uveitis	JRA, trauma	Variable	Watery	Keratitis	Injected	Small pupil

FBS: Foreign body sensation
*Positive fluorescein staining

VIII Gastrointestinal Problems

20 Abdominal Pain

Abdominal pain in children is a common and potentially emergent complaint requiring rapid assessment. The diverse locations of discomfort must be considered anatomically as well as etiologically to assist in the evaluation. (See also p. 236.)

Etiologic Considerations

Diffuse abdominal pain may be secondary to a systemic disease or a ruptured viscus producing peritonitis with rebound, guarding, and tenderness. Because of the relative absence of sensory innervation in the pelvis, disease in that region may be misleading by not producing diffuse, significant tenderness in the lower abdomen. Intestinal obstruction is accompanied by distension with high-pitched sounds and minimal rebound.

Pain may be referred. Shoulder pain may reflect diaphragmatic involvement due to basilar pneumonia, subphrenic abscess, pancreatitis, peritonitis, or injury to the spleen, gallbladder, or liver. Bilateral shoulder pain is noted if the median segment of the diaphragm is irritated. Testicular pain may reflect renal or appendiceal disease. Retroperitoneal hematoma, pancreatitis, uterine pathology, or rectal disease may cause back pain (Table 20-1).

The child's age has an impact on differential considerations. In *infants*, acute gastroenteritis and colic are common, but it is essential to exclude intussusception, volvulus, perforated viscus, and Hirschsprung's. *Preschoolers* develop pain from acute gastroenteritis, viral syndrome, urinary tract infection, trauma, appendicitis, pneumonia, constipation, and trauma. The *school-age child* frequently has acute gastroenteritis, appendicitis, urinary tract infection, trauma, functional pain, constipation, pelvic inflammatory disease (PID), ectopic pregnancy, and inflammatory bowel disease (Table 20-2).

Diagnostic Approach

1. *History* should focus on defining the acuteness and severity of the pain and possible etiologic conditions.
   - a. Describe the pain.
     - (1) Acuteness, progression, quality, location, and radiation and course pain. Potential for referred pain.
     - (2) If recurrent, events surrounding initial episode and parallel nature of pain.
     - (3) Effect of pain on normal activities.
     - (4) Response to therapeutic trials, reflecting potential etiologies such as rest, antacid.
     - (5) Factors that worsen pain.
     - (6) Change in stool pattern.
   - b. Presence of vomiting, diarrhea, weight loss, respiratory findings, dysuria, frequency, burning, vaginal discharge, dysmenorrhea, and other systemic signs or symptoms.
   - c. Concurrent events such as toilet training, stress at home or school, and trauma. Secondary gain from abdominal pain.

Table 20-1. Abdominal Pain: Anatomic Considerations

Infection/Inflammation	Congenital	Trauma	Other
Systemic			
Influenza (viral syndrome)	Sickle cell disease	Black widow spider	Constipation Functional Diabetic ketoacidosis Heavy metal Neoplasm
Abdominal Wall			
Herpes zoster	Hernia	Contusion	
Cellulitis		Hematoma	
Pulmonary			
Pneumonia		Pneumothorax	
Pleurodynia			
Gastrointestinal			
Acute gastroenteritis Mesenteric adenitis Appendicitis Gastritis/ulcer/esophagitis Peritonitis Hepatitis Pancreatitis	Meckel's diverticulum Volvulus Intussusception Hiatal hernia Hirschsprung's	Laceration liver, spleen Hematoma Perforation	Colic Ulcerative colitis Regional enteritis Neoplasm
Urinary			
Pyelonephritis Cystitis	Hydronephrosis	Renal contusion	Renal stone Wilm's tumor
Genital			
Pelvic inflammatory disease Salpingitis Epididymitis	Testicular tortion		Mittelschmerz Dysmenorrhea Ectopic pregnancy
Other			
Osteomyelitis Pelvic abscess		Fracture Herniated disc	Lactose intolerance Dissecting aortic aneurysm Epilepsy Migraine

Table 20-2. Abdominal Pain: Etiologic Considerations

Condition	Diagnostic Findings	Ancillary Data
Infection/Inflammation		
Acute gastroenteritis (Chap. 23 and 26)	Diarrhea, vomiting, diffuse abdominal pain, fever	CBC variable; fecal leukocytes
Appendicitis	Crampy abdominal pain, initially umbilical, then moving to right lower quadrant; vomiting, fever; may perforate with peritonitis	CBC elevated; UA normal; x-ray abdomen: normal, RLQ abscess, free air
Urinary tract infection (Chap. 40)	Dysuria, frequency, burning on urination; costo-vertebral angle tenderness; variable fever, toxicity	Urinalysis: white cells and bacteria; urine culture positive; CBC variable
Pelvic inflammatory disease (PID) (Chap. 28)	Lower abdominal pain; variable vaginal discharge; pelvic exam tender	CBC variable; ESR elevated; vaginal culture; ultrasound, laparoscope may be useful
Inflammatory bowel disease	Variable discomfort; abnormal stool; systemic findings	CBC normal; ESR elevated; barium enema, sigmoidoscopy diagnostic
Congenital		
Intussusception	Diffuse, severe pain, distension; variable mass, peristaltic wave; blood "currant jelly" stool; altered mental status; rare perforation, peritonitis; children < 1 year or lead point	CBC normal; x-ray abdomen: mass, obstruction and air-fluid level; barium enema diagnostic and therapeutic; sonography
Hirschsprung's disease	Distension, vomiting; failure to pass meconium in first 24 hours of life; constipated; rectal: empty ampulla, evacuation of gas and stool; rare perforation	CBC normal; barium enema: normal diameter aganglionic segment, dilated proximal segment; rectal biopsy; manometry
Meckel's diverticulum	Right lower quadrant pain, nausea, vomiting, lower GI hemorrhage; may be painless; rare perforation	CBC elevated, Hct decreased; x-ray abdomen: nondiagnostic; technetium scan positive
Volvulus	Crampy, sudden abdominal pain in lower quadrants; may be intermittent; abdomen distended, tender; rectum empty; vomiting; newborns and children 2–14 years	CBC normal; x-ray abdomen: colonic distension; barium enema diagnostic

Table 20-2. Abdominal Pain: Etiologic Considerations (*continued*)

Condition	Diagnostic Findings	Ancillary Data
Miscellaneous		
Colic (Chap. 9)	Irritable child in first 3 months of life; episodic, usually in late afternoon; otherwise normal history, physical	Therapeutic trial of reassurance, soothing rhythmic activities (rocking, wind-up swing), avoiding stimulants
Constipation (Chap. 22)	Diffuse, crampy, inconsistent abdominal pain with variable history; abdomen diffusely tender; few associated findings; may occur with toilet training	X-ray abdomen: marked stool present; trial of laxatives
Lactose intolerance	Diffuse pain with diarrhea; exam nonspecific	Trial of lactose withdrawal

2. *Physical examination* must determine the patient's hemodynamic and respiratory stability and then anatomically attempt to localize the pain.

a. Complete abdominal and rectal examination focusing on distension, bowel sounds, guarding, rebound, and tenderness. Rectal examination.

b. Pelvic examination including cultures should be done when appropriate.

c. Assessment of chest, genitalia, hernias, and other potential contributing areas.

3. *Diagnostic work-up.*

a. Laboratory.

(1) CBC and urinalysis are commonly done. Electrolytes and ESR may be useful.

(2) Other studies may include amylase, fecal leukocytes, liver function tests, pregnancy test, and peritoneal lavage.

b. Radiology.

Abdominal x-ray, barium enema, and sonography may be diagnostic. Intravenous pyelogram, upper GI series, and cholecytogram may also be contributory.

Alert: Abdominal pain may be functional but may also present with nonspecific gastrointestinal findings.

Bibliography

Brender JD, Marcuse EK, Koepsell TD, et al.: Childhood appendicitis: factors associated with perforation. Pediatrics 76:301, 1985.

Hatch EI, Jr: The acute abdomen in children. Pediatr Clin N Am 32:1151, 1985.

Johnson DC and Rice RP: The acute abdomen: plain radiographic evaluation. RadioGraphics 5:259, 1985.

Silen W: *Cope's Early Diagnosis of the Acute Abdomen* (17th ed.). New York: McGraw-Hill, 1987.

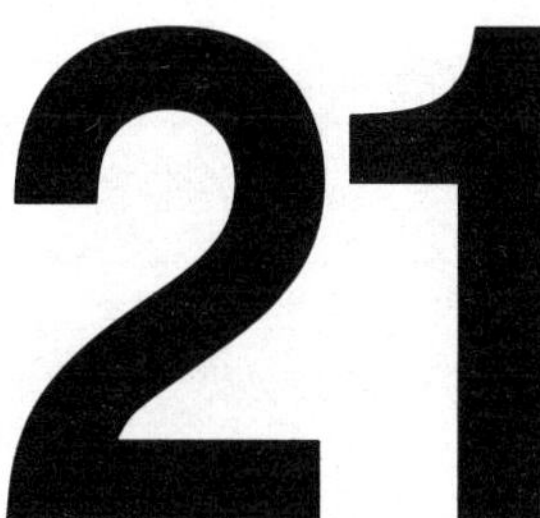

Gastrointestinal Bleeding: Hematemesis and Rectal Bleeding

Gastrointestinal bleeding, whether it be mainfested by vomiting (hematemesis) or rectal bleeding (melena), reflects infectious, inflammatory, or anatomic pathology.

The differential considerations are affected by the age of the child (Table 21-1) and the anatomical site of bleeding. Lesions *proximal to the ligament of Treitz* will usually result in nasogastric (NG) aspirates positive for blood. *Bright red* hematemesis indicates that there is little or no contact with gastric juices; it results from an active bleeding site at or above the cardia. In children it is usually caused by varices or esophagitis. Occasionally brisk duodenal or gastric bleeding may be bright red. *Coffee ground* aspirates indicate that there has been an alteration in the material by the gastric juices.

Hemoptysis must be differentiated from hematemesis, the former usually presenting with a red, frothy material mixed with sputum (Chap. 46).

The character of rectal bleeding reflects the amount and site of bleeding. Hemorrhage *proximal to the ileocecal valve* produces black, tarry stools owing to the presence of blood altered by intestinal juices (melena). *Gross blood* is generally associated with lower intestinal bleeding; rapid transit upper gastrointestinal hemorrhage may have a similar character known as hematochezia.

Medicine, food, and several other substances can produce black or red stools. Substances causing confusion include iron, large numbers of chocolate sandwich cookies, flavored gelatin, fruit juice, Kool-Aid, several antibiotics (ampicillin, lincomycin), bismuth (Pepto-Bismol), lead, licorice, charcoal, and coal.

Diagnostic Approach

The diagnostic evaluation must focus on the potential for hemodynamic instability and the site and etiology of the hemorrhage (Table 21-2).

1. *Historically*, important data relating to the urgency and differential considerations may be derived.
   a. Careful assessment of the onset, progression, character, frequency, and quality of bleeding. Associated vomiting, diarrhea, and abdominal pain.
   b. Accompanying hemodynamic instability, including dizziness and weakness.
   c. Systemic signs and symptoms.
   d. History of previous bleeding problems or family history of gastrointestinal disease.
   e. Drug history of intake of aspirin, alcohol, caustic agent, or other gastric irritants.
   f. Newborn history of umbilical vessel catheterization or necrotizing enterocolitis.
2. *Physical examination* should determine hemodynamic stability and assess the character of the bleeding.
   a. Hemodynamic stability must be assessed, including orthostatic vital signs, poor perfusion capillary refill, and altered mental status.
   b. Abdominal examination to evaluate bowel sounds, tenderness, rebound, guarding, and rectal disease.
   c. All patients with presumptive upper gastrointestinal bleeding should have a nasogastric (NG) tube inserted to determine the nature and severity of bleeding.

Table 21-1. Gastrointestinal Hemorrhage: Etiologic Considerations by Age

Infant (< 3 mo)	Toddler (< 2 yr)	Preschool (< 5 yr)	School Age (> 5 yr)
Upper Gastrointestinal Bleeding			
Swallowed blood	Esophagitis	Esophagitis	Esophagitis
Gastritis	Gastritis	Gastritis	Gastritis
Bleeding diathesis	Ulcer	Ulcer	Ulcer
Ulcer, stress	Mallory-Weiss syndrome	Esophageal varices	Esophageal varices
Pyloric stenosis	Vascular malformation	Foreign body	Mallory-Weiss syndrome
Foreign body (NG tube)	Duplication	Mallory-Weiss syndrome	Inflammatory bowel disease*
Vascular malformation		Hemophilia	Hemophilia
Duplication		Vascular malformation	Vascular malformation
Lower Gastrointestinal Bleeding			
Infection*	Infection*	Infection*	Infection*
Anal fissure	Anal fissure	Anal fissure	Inflammatory bowel disease*
Milk allergy	Milk allergy	Polyp	Ulcer
Bleeding diathesis	Intussusception*	Foreign body	Pseudomembranous enterocolitis*
Necrotizing enterocolitis*	Polyp	Intussusception*	Polyp
Meckel's diverticulum	Meckel's diverticulum	Meckel's diverticulum	Hemolytic uremic syndrome
Volvulus	Duplication	Inflammatory bowel disease	Hemorrhoid
Swallowed blood	Inflammatory bowel disease	Hemolytic uremic syndrome*	
Sepsis	Hemolytic uremic syndrome*	Henoch-Schonlein purpura*	
Peritonitis			

*Commonly associated with systemic illness involving multiple organ systems either primarily or secondarily.

Note: (1) Bleeding diathesis may include hemophilia, idiopathic thrombocytopenia pupura, vitamin K deficiency, liver dysfunction, aplastic anemia, leukemia, and disseminated intravascular coagulation.

(2) Inflammatory bowel diseases: ulcerative colitis, Crohn's disease.

Table 21-2. Hematemesis and Rectal Bleeding: Etiologic Considerations

Condition	Diagnostic Findings	Ancillary Data	Comments
Infection/Inflammation			
Acute diarrhea (Chap. 23)	Stool: variable blood; fever, diarrhea	Stool leukocytes, culture, CBC	Dietary manipulation
Gastritis	NG aspirate: coffee ground; vomiting	NG tube, upper GI series, endoscopy	Acute gastroenteritis, ASA, alcohol, caffeine, theophylline
Ulcer	NG aspirate: red/coffee ground Stool: tarry; vomiting, pain	NG tube, upper GI series, endoscopy	May be life-threatening; antacid, cimetidine
Esophagitis	NG aspirate: red/coffee ground; vomiting, retrosternal pain	Upper GI series, esophagoscopy	Hiatal hernia; chalasia, reflux
Ulcerative colitis	Stool: red/tarry; insidious weight loss	Proctoscopy, barium swallow	Multiple complications
Crohn's (regional enteritis)	Stool: red; insidious weight loss	Proctoscopy, barium swallow	Multiple complications
Anatomic			
Intussusception (Chap. 20)	Stool: "currant jelly"; abdominal pain, unstable	Hydrostatic barium enema	Life-threatening; enema or surgery
Volvulus	Stool: red/tarry; bile stained vomit, shock, abdominal pain	Barium enema	Life-threatening; surgery
Anal fissure	Stool: blood streaked; well child	Inspection	Stool softener
Polyp	Stool: red, intermittent; variable anemia	Proctoscopy, barium enema	May be inflammatory, adenoma, hemartoma
Meckel's diverticulum	Stool: red/tarry; variable stable	Pertechnetate scan	
Vascular			
Esophageal varices	NG aspirate: red, rapid Stool: tarry; cirrhosis, portal vein thrombosis	Esophagoscopy, barium swallow	
Hemangioma/hematoma/telangiectasia	Stool: red, tarry, or occult	Angiography, laparotomy	Familial (Peutz Jeghers)
Mallory-Weiss syndrome	NG aspirate: red, rapid; history, vomiting	Esophagoscopy	

Table 21-2. *(continued)*

Condition	Diagnostic Findings	Ancillary Data	Comments
Trauma			
Foreign body	Stool: red, variable; history, rectal pain	Digital exam, proctoscopy	
Blunt/penetrating trauma	NG aspirate: variable Stool: variable; reflects injury	CBC, type and cross match, radiologic studies	Reflect nature of injury
Autoimmune/Allergy			
Milk allergy (cow or soy)	Stool: red, occult; recurrent vomiting, diarrhea, colic, failure to thrive	Dietary history	
Henoch-Schonlein purpura	Stool: red/tarry; abdominal pain, arthritis, purpura, hematuria	CBC, renal function	Risk of intussusception increased
Miscellaneous			
Iron deficiency anemia (Chap. 29)	Stool: occult; pale, decreased energy	CBC, iron	Iron supplementation
Swallowed blood	Stool: occult; otherwise well	CBC, Apt test	Newborn (maternal blood), epistaxis

d. Patients with suspected lower intestinal bleeding should have a rectal examination and assessment for gross and occult blood.

3. *Diagnostic work-up.*

a. Laboratory.

(1) Blood may be identified with guaiac, benzidine, or benzidine-derivative impregnated test pads (Hemoccult, Hamatest), the latter being the most readily available and popular technique. A thin smear of stool is applied to a pad. The application of a hydrogen peroxide developer results in a blue discoloration in the presence of blood.

(a) False positives may be obtained due to red meat, iron, and vegetables (broccoli and turnips) while false negatives result from a low pH of the fluid (gastric aspirate), breakdown of hemoglobin by gut flora, and interfering medications such as vitamin C. The technique is therefore unreliable in the assessment of gastric contents.

(b) Swallowed maternal blood may be identified by performing the Apt test. One part of gastric contents or stool is mixed with five parts of water and centrifuged. Add 0.1 ml of 0.2 N sodium hydroxide to the supernatant fluid. A pink color developing in 2–5 minutes indicates fetal hemoglobin and a brown color signifies adult hemoglobin.

(2) Baseline screening studies are indicated following confirmation of hemorrhage including a CBC, platelets, and coagulation tests (PT, PTT, and bleeding time) (see Chap. 30).

(3) Type and cross match should be sent in hemodynamically unstable patients.

(4) Specific evaluation of stool including fecal leukocytes, bacterial culture, and ova and parasites as indicated.

(5) Endoscopic examination should reflect the diagnostic conditions and include gastroduodenoscopy for upper gastrointestinal bleeding and proctosigmoidoscopy for lower GI bleeding.

(6) Radiologic examination should include an upper gastrointestinal tract study or barium enema for specific presentations. Air contrast barium enemas are particularly useful in evaluating mucosal lesions.

Alert: Gastrointestinal bleeding may cause hemodynamic instability that must be assessed and treated before diagnostic evaluation is initiated.

Bibliography

Hyams JS, Leichtner AM, Schwartz AN: Recent advances in diagnosis and treatment of gastrointestinal hemorrhage in infants and children. J Pediatr 106:1, 1985.

Jenkins HR, Pincott JR, Soothill JF, et al.: Food allergy: the major cause of infantile colitis. Arch Dis Child 59:326, 1984.

Lifton LJ, Kneiser J: False-positive stool occult blood tests caused by iron preparations. Gastroenterology 83:860, 1982.

Steer ML and Silen W: Diagnostic procedures in gastrointestinal hemorrhage. N Engl J Med 309:646, 1983.

22 Constipation

Children having difficulty with bowel movements may be constipated if there is an abnormality in the character of the stool as well as if there is an abnormality in its frequency. In general, constipation is present when stools are hard, infrequent, and painful to pass. In the presence of fecal impaction, stools may become watery to allow passage past the relative obstruction caused by the impaction. Elimination patterns reflect familial, cultural, social, dietary, and anatomical factors. Determination of a change in stool patterns is essential.

Stooling is initially a reflex act; peristaltic movement associated with relaxation of the internal and external anal sphincters leads to defecation. Thereafter, voluntary control develops over the external anal sphincter.

Normal stool patterns vary with age and diet. Ninety-five percent of neonates pass meconium in the first 24 hours of life. During the first 3–4 days of life, greenish-black, odorless, and thick meconium stools are common. Subsequently, transitional, green-brown, slimy stools are passed up to 8 times per day although some babies may go as long as 24 hours without passing stools. Milk stools develop after a week. Breast-fed babies have pasty, light yellow stools while formula fed children have firm, yellow stools. The frequency decreases with some children having stools every 2–3 days although more commonly there are one to two stools per day. Older children have stools reflecting diet and eating habits.

Constipation is often associated with the process of toilet training, particularly when frustration and resistance are encountered. It is not uncommon for boys to remain untrained after 3 or 4 years of age. (See also Chap. 7 and p. 248.)

Etiologic Considerations

The classification reflects the intactness of peristaltic action including mass peristaltic movement of the colon, relaxation of the anal sphincters, contraction of voluntary muscles, and interference of autonomic and cortical control of defecation.

There is often an interplay of multiple psychologic, physiologic, and environmental factors (Table 22-1). Many patients will have intermittent chronic abdominal pain, often of a crampy nature.

Diagnostic Approach

1. *History* should focus on the changing pattern of the stool and whether the constipation has associated signs and symptoms.
   a. Characteristics of the stool including the frequency, consistency, color, odor, and previous patterns.
   b. Associated problems focusing on anorexia, tenesmus, and abdominal pain. The pain may be crampy or constant. Fecal soiling (encopresis) should be discussed.
   c. Previous stooling pattern and family history of similar problems.
   d. Evaluation of personal and family stresses and maternal and paternal interaction with the child.

Table 22-1. Constipation: Etiologic Considerations

Condition	Impairment	Comments
Dietary		
Lack of fecal bulk	Stimulus to peristalsis	Minimal roughage intake; excessive use of enemas, laxatives
Excessive cow's milk intake	Peristalsis	Resultant hard stools; also early introduction to cereals, yellow vegetables
Psychiatric		
Difficult toilet training, retention, resistance, holding, psychopathology, depression, anxiety	Spinal arc	Resistance or problematic training, voluntary retention, or habit; often associated with abdominal pain; encopresis may develop, impairing cortical function (Chap. 7)
Congenital		
Intestinal atresia Imperforate anus Meconium plug Peritonitis, ileus	Mechanical obstruction, peristalsis	Fecal stream blocked; variety of other acute, chronic, acquired, and congenital anatomical lesions
Hirschsprung's disease	Peristalsis	Aganglionic megacolon with subsegmental absence of ganglion; newborn; intestinal obstruction, delayed meconium passage; rectum-empty ampulla
Myelomeningocele	Spinal arc	Other neurologic conditions may be causative
Anal stenosis	Relaxation of anal sphincter	Newborn/infancy
Trauma		
Anal fissure	Relaxation of anal sphincter	Small tears of the anus, often accompanied by blood streaking of the stools and pain
Intoxication		
Excessive enemas, suppositories	Stimulus to peristalsis	Decreases sensitivity to normal reflexes
Excessive use antihistamines, diuretics, narcotics, calcium channel blockers	Peristalsis	Use reduces peristalsis; excessive use may lead to impaction
Metabolic/Endocrine		
Hypothyroidism Hypercalcemia Hypokalemia	Peristalsis	Associated clinical signs and symptoms

e. Assessment of diet and response to previous dietary manipulation. In babies, changes of diet may have included addition of 1–2 teaspoons of Karo syrup to each bottle. In infants, apricots, pears, and other fruits may be used. Older children should be assessed for intake of roughage, such as fruits and vegetables and particularly prunes, figs, raisins, beans, celery, and lettuce. Bran and other natural laxatives such as Maltsupex may have already been tried.
f. Utilization of enemas and suppositories.
g. Resistance to toilet training.
h. Newborn stooling pattern including characteristics of first stool, frequency, etc.

2. *Physical examination* normally focuses on the abdomen and rectum.
   a. A palpable, cylindric mass may be demonstrated in the abdomen.
   b. Abdomen may have variable bowel sounds. Distension and minimal, diffuse tenderness are not uncommon.
   c. Rectal examination determining amount and character of stool, presence of blood (mixed, streaking), tone.
   d. Vital signs, including orthostatics, should be documented.
3. *Diagnostic work-up* should include:
   a. Laboratory.
      (1) Complete blood count with differential.
      (2) Assessment of stool for blood.
      (3) Rarely, abdominal x-ray film may demonstrate retained stool that is granular or rock-like in appearance.
      (4) Rectal monometry is diagnostic of aganglionoic megacolon. Rectal biopsy or barium enema may be useful.
   b. Therapeutic trial may consist of the following:
      (1) Alteration of diet as discussed above to increase roughage and osmotic load.
      (2) Milk laxatives.
         (a) Maltsupex.
         (b) Senta syrup (Senokot), ¼ teaspoon per day slowly.
      (3) With marked retention, initial clearance may be attempted using pediatric Fleets enemas twice, followed by Dulcolax suppositories twice with Discodyl tablets orally. Mineral oil, 1–6 tablespoons per day, may be ultimately required.

Alert: Constipation is usually functional in nature, reflecting such stresses as toilet training or environmental changes but may occur due to a number of organic conditions that should be excluded.

Bibliography

Fleisher DR: Diagnosis and treatment of disorders of defecation in children. Pediatr Ann 5:700, 1976.

Leoning-Baucke V, Cruikshank B, and Savage C: Defecation dynamics and behavioral profiles in encopretic children. Pediatrics 80:672, 1987.

23 Diarrhea

Diarrhea relates to a loosening of stool consistency, commonly associated with an increase in frequency. Diarrhea refers to a change in an individual's usual pattern.

Large volumes of fluid are handled by the gastrointestinal tract, primarily following osmotic gradients created by electrolytes and other osmotically active substances (glucose, amino acids) in a passive manner. Alterations in this balance may result in a number of pathologic processes: osmotic diarrhea, whereby absorbable, osmotically active substances are osmotically drawn into the intestinal lumen; secretory diarrhea, resulting from an electrolyte secretory process into the lumen; and motility problems with rapid or impaired intestinal transit times (Table 23-1). (See also p. 255.)

Etiologic Considerations

Acute diarrhea is primarily infectious in origin, rarely reflecting extraperitoneal or peritoneal irritation, pneumonia, otitis media, or urinary tract infection. Malabsorption, mechanical abnormalities, or systemic disease can also be contributory.

In differentiating contributing *acute* conditions, important characteristics include the acuteness of the diarrhea, fever, and presence of blood. Bloody diarrhea in febrile children commonly has an infectious origin while diarrhea without blood may have a viral etiology or an extraintestinal cause. Bacterial gastroenteritis is more likely in children with a history of blood in the stool in combination with either a fever > 38°C or at least ten stools in 14 hours. Afebrile children with bloody diarrhea must have intussusception, pseudomembranous colitis, or hemolytic uremic syndrome excluded; nonbloody diarrhea usually has a noninfectious origin related to malabsorption, drugs, and so on.

In the case of *chronic diarrhea*, consider inflammatory bowel disease, irritable bowel syndrome, post-infectious malabsorption, malabsorption, secretory disorders secondary to hormone or toxin secretion, anatomic abnormality (especially Hirschsprung's disease), parasites, systemic disease, immunodeficiency, cystic fibrosis, overfeeding, antibiotics, toxins, and disaccharide, monosaccharide, or lactase deficiency.

See also Chap. 26.

Diagnostic Approach

1. *History* should focus on the changing stooling pattern, rapidity of onset, and associated findings after a determination that there is no hemodynamic instability associated with dizziness or malaise, for example.
   - **a.** Stool pattern: consistency, mucous, blood, frequency, and response to food intake.
   - **b.** Onset, progression and response to alterations in diet such as elimination of specific groups or initiation of clear liquids, medications, or other measures.
   - **c.** Associated signs and symptoms including fever, rash, arthralgia.
   - **d.** Reoccurrence and exposures.
   - **e.** Urine output.

Table 23-1. Acute Diarrhea: Etiologic Considerations

Condition	Diagnostic Findings	Comments
Infection		
Acute gastroenteritis		
Viral	Loose stools, rare blood, WBCs; respiratory symptoms; acute onset; electron microscopy, ELISA rotavirus	Rotavirus, Norwalk agent, enterovirus
Bacterial	Loose, watery stool, variable blood, WBCs (methylene blue), culture; toxic, vomiting, fever, seizure *(Shigella)*, abdominal pain	*Shigella, salmonella*, campylobacter, *vibrio*
Parasite	Variable stool pattern; chronic; weight loss; ova and parasite	*Giardia lamblia, Entamoeba histolytica*
Post-infectious malabsorption	Water loss, rare blood in stool; resolving infectious gastroenteritis; reducing substance, pH < 5 in stool	Lactose intolerance, excessive bile salts
Acute appendicitis/ peritonitis	Variable stool; rebound, guarding, toxicity	Multiple underlying problems
Extra-gastrointestinal-respiratory, urinary tract, etc.	Reflects underlying pathology	
Autoimmune/Allergic		
Ulcerative colitis	Mucousy stool with PMNs, blood; tenesmus, urgency, abdominal pain, fever, weight loss, systemic (arthritis, etc.); sigmoidoscopy, barium enema; elevated ESR	10–19-year-old peak; insidious
Regional enteritis (Crohn's)	Bloody, watery stool; abdominal pain, fever, perianal disease; sigmoidoscopy, barium enema; elevated ESR	Teenagers
Milk allergy	Bloody, watery stool; vomiting, anemia	Dietary elimination; lactose intolerance
Gluten sensitivity (celiac disease)	Bulky, pale, frothy stool; failure to thrive, vomiting, abdominal pain; biopsy	Dietary elimination; onset reflects age introduction gluten (wheat, rye, oats)

Table 23-1. *(continued)*

Condition	Diagnostic Findings	Comments
Psychosomatic		
Fear/anxiety	Loose stool; response to recent stress	Stress reduction technique
Fecal impaction (encopresis) (Chap. 7)	Loose, watery stool; abdominal pain; constipation	Overflow incontinence
Congenital		
Cystic fibrosis	Fatty, bulky, foul-smelling stool; failure to thrive, pulmonary disease; sweat test	Congenital; variable penetrance
Hirschsprung's disease	Green, watery, foul-smelling stool; abdominal distension, fever, poor growth; rectal biopsy, barium enema	
Intussusception (Chap. 20)	Bloody stool; abdominal pain with abrupt onset; barium enema	
Miscellaneous		
Irritable bowel syndrome	Watery, mucousy stool, commonly after intake food; normal growth	Therapeutic trial of reducing frequency food; no spicy, hot, cold foods
Intoxication	Loose stools; variable findings	Antibiotics, iron, antimetabolites; pseudomembranous colitis (*C. difficile*)
Hyperthyroidism	Loose stools; systemic findings; thyroid studies	
Neoplasm	Watery stool; variable findings	Lymphoma, carcinoma, neuroblastoma, Zollinger Ellison syndrome

2. *Physical examination* should initially focus on hemodynamic stability, hydration status, and alertness.
Abdominal and rectal examination to assess associated findings with stool examined for blood. Repeated examinations may be useful.

3. *Diagnostic work-up.*

a. Laboratory must assess etiologic considerations and current stability.

(1) Hydration status including BUN, Na^+, Cl^-, K^+, HCO_3^-, urine specific gravity.

(2) Stool polys (methylene blue), culture, rotavirus examination, ova and parasites.

(3) CBC with differential may be helpful.

(4) Sigmoidoscopy or rectal biopsy are rarely required but may be helpful in evaluation of chronic diarrhea.

b. Radiologic examination may include barium enema in specific circumstances.

Alert: Diarrhea is often associated with abnormal fluid losses requiring fluid resuscitation.

Bibliography

Barkin RM: Acute infectious diarrheal disease in children. J Emerg Med 3:1, 1985.

DeWitt TG, Humphrey KF, McCarthy P: Clinical predictors of acute bacterial diarrhea in young children. Pediatrics 76:551, 1985.

Kapikian AZ, Whakin H, Whatt RG, et al.: Human reovirus-like agent as the major pathogen associated with "winter" gastroenteritis in hospitalized infants and young children. N Engl J Med 294:965, 1976.

Listernick R, Sieseri E, and Davis AT: Outpatient oral rehydration in the United States. Am J Dis Child 140:211, 1986.

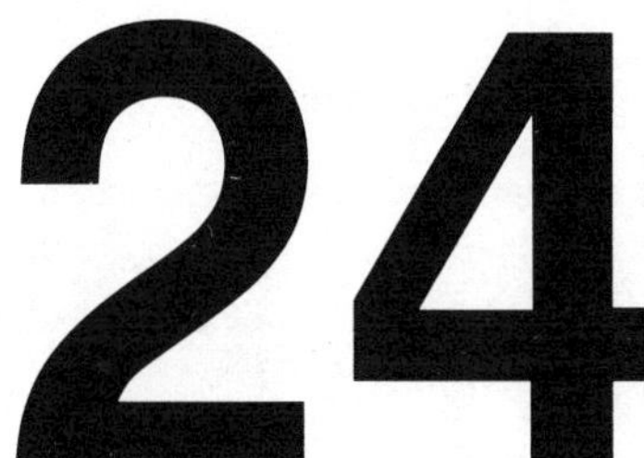

Dysphagia

Difficulty swallowing is uncommon in children and may result from pharyngeal, laryngeal, or esophageal lesions. Dysphagia results from *anatomic obstruction or compression* or a *physiologic dysfunction* of the neuromuscular mechanism of swallowing (Table 24-1).

Etiologic Considerations

Preesophageal problems are often accompanied by systemic illness such as myasthenia gravis. Motor disturbances producing esophageal dysphagia cause problems with solids and liquids while obstructive disease primarily causes dysphagia for solids only.

Diagnostic Approach

1. *Historically*, it is often possible to delineate the probable mechanism and level of dysfunction.
   a. Rapidity of onset and recurrence; improving or progressing; congenital or acquired.
   b. Accompanying pain, discomfort, vomiting.
   c. Difficulty with liquids or solids.
   d. Systemic signs and symptoms.
2. *Physical examination* should assess if evidence of systemic signs and symptoms exist while examining the pharynx for evidence of disease.
3. *Diagnostic work-up* requires radiologic or endoscopic examination.
   a. Laboratory.
      (1) Cultures, electrolytes, calcium, magnesium, drug levels, cerebrospinal fluid.
      (2) Manometry to measure upper and lower esophageal pressures and the peristaltic wave. Esophageal pH.
      (3) Fiberoptic esophagoscopy to evaluate esophagitis, reflux, mass lesions, function.
   b. Radiology.
      (1) Barium swallow and fluoroscopy to exclude narrowing, stricture, and foreign body and examine the swallowing mechanism.
      (2) Lateral neck film to evaluate neck mass.
      (3) CT scan.
   c. Therapeutic trial should include the tensilon (endrophonium) trial.

Alert: Although usually an upper airway or esophageal problem, systemic conditions must be excluded. Dehydration may accompany the condition.

Table 24-1. Dysphagia: Physiologic and Etiologic Considerations

	Primary Mechanism		
	Obstruction/ Compressive (mechanical)	Physiologic Dysfunction (motor)	Diagnostic Findings
Infection/Inflammatory			
Tonsillitis (Chap. 17)	+		Sore throat, fever; group A strep, virus, mononucleosis
Stomatitis	+		Sore throat, ulcer; aphthous, herpes
Peritonsillar abscess	+		Asymmetrical tonsils, abscess, lateral neck
Retropharyngeal abscess	+		Swelling, tenderness, lateral neck
Epiglottitis, croup (Chap. 46)	+		Stridor, progressive, difficulty breathing, visualize epiglottis
Botulism, rabies, polio		+	Cranial nerve abnormality, rapid onset, exposure, diplopia
Chalasia, gastroesophageal reflux, esophagitis, hiatal hernia (Chap. 26)		+	Regurgitation, retrosternal pain, esophageal pH low
Intoxication			
Caustic ingestion	+	+	History of ingestion, burning; esophagoscopy
Phenothiazine		+	Diplopia, ataxia
Congenital			
Cleft palate	+		Early onset pain, vomiting
Macroglossia	+		
Esophageal web, atresia	+		
Familiar dysautonomia		+	Familial; aspiration
Vascular ring, aneurysm	+		

Psychiatric			
Globus hystericus		+	Spasm pharynx (lump in throat)
Miscellaneous			
Foreign body	+		History, acute onset
Neuromuscular disease		+	Accompanying signs, symptoms
Guillain-Barre			
Myasthenia gravis			
Brain damage		+	Variable retardation
Hypothyroidism, goiter, thyroiditis	+	+	Neck mass, variable hypotonia
Neoplasm (carcinoma, Hodgkin's disease)	+		Systemic signs, symptoms

Bibliography

Pope CE: Motor disorders of the esophagus. Postgrad Med 61:155, 1977.

Werlin SL, Dodds WJ, Hogan WJ, et al.: Mechanisms of gastroesophageal reflux in children. J Pediatr 97:244, 1980.

25 Hepatosplenomegaly

Hepatic or splenic enlargement may be associated or be present independently. Apparent enlargement of the liver may be confirmed by percussion. The liver edge is commonly palpable in newborns with the mean liver span increasing from 7 cm at 5 years of age to 9 cm by 12 years.

The spleen is palpable in as many as 30% of infants, decreasing to 10% by 1 year of age and to 1% in children and adolescents.

Etiologic Considerations

Commonly hepatic or splenic enlargement may be due to infection, anemia and hemolytic processes, passive congestion from cardiac failure, metabolic diseases, and infiltrative disease associated with neoplasm or congenital metabolic conditions (Table 25-1). Hepatomegaly is a cardinal sign of right side heart failure or portal hypertension.

Diagnostic Approach

1. *History* should focus on systemic illness and findings.
   - **a.** Family history of hypoglycemia, metabolic disease, hepatosplenomegaly.
   - **b.** Evidence of hypoglycemia or mental and neurologic deterioration. Abnormal growth and development.
   - **c.** Cardiac history evaluating shortness of breath, underlying infection, and exposure to parasitic disease or ingestion.
   - **d.** Complications in newborn period.
2. *Physical examination*.
   - **a.** Focus on growth pattern and systemic illness, such as recurrent infection, poor diet, malnutrition, protuberant abdomen, purpura, and evidence of bleeding.
   - **b.** Examination of the liver and spleen should define their size, consistency (hardness and smoothness), tenderness.
   - **c.** Careful neurological examination.
3. *Diagnostic work-up*.
   - **a.** Laboratory assessment must be broad.
     - **(1)** Glucose, electrolytes, urinalysis.
     - **(2)** Urine for mucopolysaccharides.
     - **(3)** Liver biopsy and routine evaluation. Additionally, enzyme assay of biopsy specimen as well as of culture skin fibroblasts and peripheral leukocytes.
   - **b.** Radiologic studies including a chest x-ray, bone, and so on, as indicated.

Table 25-1. Hepatosplenomegaly: Etiologic Considerations

Conditions	Diagnostic Findings	Comments
Hepatitis	Acute or chronic disease with systemic illness, abnormal liver functions, systemic illness; variable splenic enlargement	Multiple viral cause: hepatitis, infectious mononucleosis; congenital: microcephaly, petechiae (also rubella, CMV, toxoplasmosis, etc.); rare fungal, mycobacterium
Sepsis	Hypotension, insidious or acute onset of multiple organ failure	Multiple etiologies; life-threatening
Parasitic illness Malaria, amebiasis, visceral larval migrans, liver fluke	Multiple findings and specific evaluation, hepatosplenomegaly	Exposure and epidemiology should determine potential etiologies
Juvenile rheumatoid arthriitis, SLE, inflammatory bowel	Multiple presentations	Autoimmune disease
Metabolic		
Galactosemia	Normal at birth; vomiting, diarrhea, jaundice, hepatosplenomegaly, failure to thrive, cataracts	Often die of sepsis
Mycopolysaccharidoses		
Type I – Hurler	Coarse features, macrocephaly, hirsutism, hepatosplenomegaly, mental deterioration	
Type II – Hunter	Stiff joints, dwarfism, less coarse features, hepatosplenomegaly	
Type III – Sanfilippo	Coarse features, minimal splenomegaly, mental retardation	Onset at 1–3 years
Type IV – Maroteaux-Lamy	Coarse features, stiff joint, cloudy cornea, hepatosplenomegaly	

Glycogen Storage Disease		
Type I—Von Gierke	Protuberant abdomen, hepatomegaly (smooth), splenomegaly, cardiomegaly absent; hypoglycemia, acidosis; short stature, doll-like face	
Type II—Pompe	Hypotonia, decreased reflexes develop in infancy; cardiac failure, hepatomegaly	
Type III—Forbes	Fasting hypoglycemia, hyperlipidemia; hepatomegaly, failure to thrive	
Type IV—Andersen	Hepatomegaly (nodular), splenomegaly; cirrhosis, portal hypertension	
Type V—Hers Lipid Storage Disease	Hepatomegaly, growth failure	
Gaucher Disease	Splenomegaly and later hepatomegaly; mental deterioration, patchy-brown or yellow discoloration; bony lesion	
Neimann-Pick	Hepatosplenomegaly, mental deterioration; fundus: cherry-red spot; foam cells in bone marrow	Onset at 6 months to 5 years
Gangliosidoses	Coarse features; progressive features	
Mucolipodoses	Coarse features; progressive mental deterioration, hepatomegaly; splenomegaly (I, II, mannosidosis)	
Metachromatic leukodystrophy	Hepatosplenomegaly; mental deterioration	
Wolman Disease	Hepatosplenomegaly; failure to thrive; diarrhea; calcified adrenal gland	
Alpha 1-antitrypsin disease	Cholestatic disease (jaundice, hepatosplenomegaly); anicteric hepatitis, cirrhosis	

Table 25-1. Hepatosplenomegaly: Etiologic Considerations (*continued*)

Conditions	Diagnostic Findings	Comments
Vascular		
Congestive heart failure	Insidious or rapid onset of shortness of breath, hepatomegaly	Multiple cardiac and noncardiac etiologies
Hemangioma, varices	Variable hepatosplenomegaly; CT and angiography diagnostic	
Other		
Isoimmunization disorders	Anemia, congestive heart failure; hepatosplenomegaly	Multiple etiologies; newborn
Neoplasm	Variable findings	Hepatoblastoma, carcinoma, leukemia
Cirrhosis	Liver failure	Multiple etiologies
Intoxication	Hepatocellular injury or cholestasis; hepatomegaly	Phenobarbital, hydantoin, acetaminophen, steroid

Bibliography

Gryboski J, Walker A: *Gastrointestinal Problems in the Infant* (2nd ed.). Philadelphia: Saunders, 1983.

Lawson EE, Grand RJ, Neff RK, et al.: Clinical estimation of liver span in infants and children. Am J Dis Child 132:474, 1978.

Walker WA and Mathis RK: Hepatomegaly, an approach to differential diagnosis. Pediat Clin North Am 22:929, 1975.

26 Vomiting

Vomiting is a coordinated event produced by increased intragastric pressure from the contraction of the abdominal wall musculature, lowering of the diaphragm, and closure of the gastric pylorus and glottis. The medullary vomiting center coordinates vomiting, the stimuli arising from pelvic and abdominal viscera, peritoneum, genitourinary tract, pharynx, labyrinth, and heart as well as the chemoreceptor trigger zone. This separate site is responsive to drugs such as digitalis, metabolic abnormalities, and other systemic dysfunction.

Regurgitation may sometimes be confused with vomiting but has a different physiology. It is due to reflux of gastric contents into the esophagus and mouth and may be a developmental process known as *chalasia* or esophageal or neurological disease.

(See also p. 279.)

Etiologic Considerations

Important differential features include the age of the child, evidence of obstruction, and evidence of extra-abdominal conditions. The nature of the vomiting may assist in differentiating contributing conditions (Table 26-1).

1. Undigested food suggests an esophageal lesion at or above the cardia.
2. Nonbilious vomiting results from lesions proximal to the pylorus.
3. Bilious vomiting, especially associated with the first vomitus, usually involves obstruction beyond the ampulla of Vater (in the second portion of the duodenum) or may result from an adynamic ileus secondary to sepsis, significant other infection, or serious underlying disease. In older children, persistent vomiting may lead to reflux of bile from the duodenum into the stomach leading to bilious vomiting without obstruction. Bile turns green on exposure to air.
4. A fecal odor in the vomitus occurs with peritonitis or a lower obstruction.

Also see Chap. 23.

Diagnostic Approach

1. *Historical* data is essential in determining the child's age and the nature of the vomiting.
   a. Age and previous episodes of vomiting; family history of congenital problems.
   b. Nature of the vomiting: color, composition, bilious, fecal odor, digested or undigested material, relationship to eating and position, onset, progression, projectile.
   c. Associated gastrointestinal findings including diarrhea, abdominal discomfort, distention, tenderness, rebound, and guarding.
   d. Feeding techniques.
   e. Drug, trauma, and pregnancy history.
   f. Perinatal events and exposures.
   g. Other signs and symptoms including hemodynamic and mental stability, associated conditions, mentation, headache, and fever.

Table 26-1. Vomiting: Etiologic Categories by Age

	Gastrointestinal	Other
Newborn	Gastroesophageal reflux Obstructive anomalies Intestinal stenosis Meconium ileus/plug Imperforate anus Hirschsprung's disease Necrotizing enterocolitis Cow's milk allergy	Neurologic: hydrocephalus, cerebral edema Renal: obstruction, failure Infection: sepsis, meningitis Metabolic: inborn error of metabolism, congenital adrenal hyperplasia
Infant	Gastroesophageal reflux Gastroenteritis Obstruction Pyloric stenosis Malrotation Intussusception Incarcerated hernia Hirschsprung's disease Peritonitis, appendicitis Acquired esophageal disorder	Neurologic: hydrocephalus, cerebral edema, brain tumor Renal: obstruction, failure Infection: sepsis, meningitis, urinary tract infection, otitis media, hepatitis, cough Metabolic: inborn error of metabolism, galactosemia, fructose intolerance, adrenal failure Overdose: digitalis, theophylline
Older Children	Gastroenteritis Obstruction Esophageal stricture Malrotation Foreign body Intussusception Hirschsprung's disease Peptic ulcer disease Peritonitis, appendicitis Pancreatitis	Neurologic: brain tumor, migraine, motion sickness Renal: obstruction, failure Infection: sepsis, meningitis, urinary tract infection, hepatitis, postnasal drip, cough Metabolic: diabetic ketoacidosis, adrenal insufficiency Overdose: digitalis, theophylline Pregnancy Psychogenic

2. *Physical examination* must assess toxicity and hydration status. Systemic illness and hemodynamic stability must be assessed, often requiring emergent intervention (Table 26-2).
   a. Abdominal examination including palpation and auscultation. Rectal evaluation, including hematest.
   b. Other contributing or predisposing findings including neurological status, respiratory tract, urinary, or nervous system infection or recent trauma.
3. *Diagnostic work-up.*
   a. Laboratory evaluation should assist in the evaluation of the vomitus.
      (1) Vomitus: color, bile, blood, digested material.
      (2) CBC if infectious or need to assess Hct. Hydration status if necessary including lytes and specific gravity of urine.
      (3) Blood studies as indicated, including urine for amino and organic acids, ABG, liver functions, glucose, ketones, and so on.
      (4) Urinalysis to exclude infection or renal failure.
      (5) Endoscopy, manometry, and pH studies as indicated.
   b. Radiologic studies to assess GI function.
      (1) Barium swallow or UGI studies to evaluate intestinal integrity and swallowing mechanism.
      (2) CT scan looking for CNS or abdominal abnormalities.
   c. Therapeutic trials may be useful in the assessment.
      (1) Antacids for inflammatory processes.

Table 26-2. Vomiting: Etiologic Considerations

Condition	Diagnostic Findings	Comments
Infection/Inflammation		
Acute gastroenteritis (see Chap. 23 and 26)	Acute onset diarrhea, vomiting, nausea, fever; stool variable blood, PMNs, mucous; variable dehydration	Assess hydration status; trial of NPO or clear liquids
Hepatitis	Systemic illness; liver tenderness, icterus, abnormal liver functions	Infectious: viral, mononucleosis
Peritonitis (Chap. 20) Appendicitis Cholecystitis Pancreatitis	Systemic illness; diffuse abdominal tenderness, ileus, variable rebound, guarding; elevated WBC, ultrasound, plain film, etc.	Evaluate underlying condition; surgical evaluation
Esophagitis/gastritis	Epigastric or substernal pain; reflux; variable coffee ground vomitus; Hct	Barium swallow or endoscopic evaluation; trial antacids
Extragastrointestinal Posterior nasal drip/posttussive	Vomiting worse when lying down, rhinorrhea; following vigorous coughing (Chap. 44)	Evaluate underlying condition; trial of decongestant or cough suppressant
Otitis media	Ear pain, fever, rhinorrhea	Treat
Cystitis/pyelonephritis (Chap. 40)	Dysuria, frequency, burning; variable fever, CVA tenderness	Responds to antibiotics
Meningitis (Chap. 32)	Listless, toxic, variable focal findings; lumbar puncture; CT, if question increased pressure	Life-threatening; may accompany other infection
Congenital		
Gastrointestinal obstruction/band/stenosis Malrotation Volvulus Intussusception	Obstructive pattern, often beginning as newborn or in infancy; if proximal to ampulla of Vater, distension epigastrium or LUQ and gastric peristaltic wave; if distal to ampulla of Vater, vomitus contains bile and distension generalized; abdominal flat plate, contrast study	Potentially life-threatening; evaluate hydration; trial of decompression; surgical consultation

Pyloric stenosis	Regurgitation progressing to vomiting (often projectile); insidious; palpable olive-sized tumor in RUQ; gastric peristaltic wave; poor weight gain; barium swallow or ultrasound	Usually male, 4–6 weeks of age; evaluate hydration; surgical consultation
Hydrocephalus	Excessive head circumference growth; irritability, headache, bulging fontanelle; CT scan	Variable underlying pathology; neurosurgical consult
Trauma (Chap. 47)		
Concussion Subdural hematoma Epidural hematoma Subarachnoid hemorrhage	Trauma, followed by altered mental status; evidence of increased intracranial pressure; variable focal findings; seizures; CT scan	Potentially life-threatening; neurosurgical consultation
Intramural hematoma	Blunt trauma; abdominal tenderness, nausea, ileus, bilous vomiting; upper GI series, CT scan	Often associated with seat belt injury; may also rupture viscus
Endocrine/Metabolic		
Acidosis	Rapid, deep breathing; ABG	Define etiology
Diabetic ketoacidosis	Kussmaul's breathing; abdominal pain; history of diabetes; glucose, ketones, ABG	Define predisposing illness
Inborn errors of metabolism	Early onset vomiting, acidosis; progressive deterioration, poor growth, developmental delay; urine and blood amino and organic acids	Exacerbated by acute illness; metabolic consultation
Adrenal failure	Acute or insidious nausea, weakness, dehydration, fatigue; K^+ elevated, Na^+ decreased; urinary steroids	Acquired; congenital adrenogenital syndrome

Table 26-2. Vomiting: Etiologic Considerations (*continued*)

Condition	Diagnostic Findings	Comments
Miscellaneous		
Improper feeding Chalasia	Associated with regurgitation; occurs after feeding; vomited material is undigested; child well with good growth; rarely UGI study to exclude pathology	Improper position, overfeeding; overanxious parent; trial of slow, careful, prone upright feeding; improves by 6 months
Intoxication	Local irritation esophagus or stomach; central effect	Alkali burn, aspirin, digitalis, iron, lead
Migraine headache (Chap. 34)	Unilateral, throbbing headache; aura, family history	Trial of analgesia, steroids, ergotamine
Epilepsy	Aura or seizure; EEG	Trial anticonvulsants
Pregnancy	First trimester nausea, discomfort; pregnancy test	Increased intraabdominal pressure
Attention getting Hysteria Hyperventilation	Inconsistent history or anxiety; may be related to other psychosomatic symptoms	Related to stress; exclude organic causes
Hyperthermia	Abnormal mental status; variable cramps, fever, dehydration; lytes	Exposure to excessive heat
Neoplasm	Related to location, type, extent	Rare in children

(2) Support and altered feeding techniques may be curative.
Alert: Although vomiting is usually self-limited, it may lead to dehydration or be associated with life-threatening conditions.

Bibliography

Forman SJ, Filer LJ, Anderson TA, et al.: Recommendations for feeding normal infants. Pediatrics 73:52, 1979.

Hargrove CB, Ulshen MH, and Shub MD: Upper gastrointestinal endoscopy in infants: diagnostic usefulness and safety. Pediatrics 74:828, 1984.

Silverman A, Roy CC: *Pediatric Clinical Gastroenterology* (3rd ed.). St. Louis: CV Mosby, 1983.

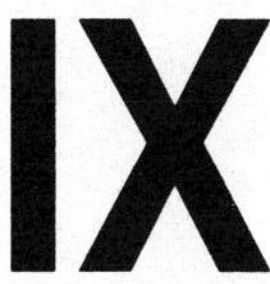

IX Gynecologic Problems

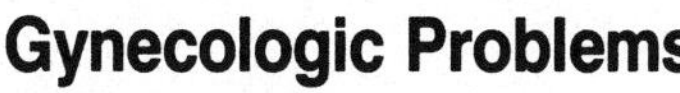

27 Vaginal Bleeding

Vaginal bleeding in prepubescent girls results from localized vaginal or uterine pathology; following puberty, hypothalamic-pituitary problems, complications of pregnancy, and local problems may be causative (Table 27-1).

Etiologic Considerations

Prepubertal children can develop vaginal bleeding due to a variety of conditions. Vulvovaginal infection, trauma, excoriation, foreign body, tumors, condyloma, and bleeding diathesis have been implicated. Neonates may have a blood tinged discharge due to withdrawal of circulating maternal estrogens.

Following *puberty*, normal periods are about 28 days apart (measured from the first day of one period to the first day of the next) and last 6 days or less. Bleeding is excessive when it increases over the normal pattern; bleeding generally does not exceed 6 pads or 10 tampons. Menstrual irregularity is frequent during the first year following menarche and as many as 20% of teenagers continue this pattern for up to 5 years.

Dysfunctional uterine bleeding may be caused by endocrine disorders, infection, weight change, and psychiatric stress. Anovulatory cycles commonly accompany dysfunctional bleeding in which the bleeding is scanty, watery, and irregular.

Also see Chap. 28.

Diagnostic Approach

1. *History* should focus on gynecologic problems and systemic illness.
   - **a.** Menstrual history and sexual development. Exposure to diethylstilbestrol in utero.
   - **b.** Sexual pattern including frequency, recent trauma, likelihood of abuse, foreign body. Last menstrual period, intercourse in interim and possibility of pregnancy. Exposure to venereal disease.
   - **c.** Endocrine history, weight change, potential ingestion, medications, bleeding problems, systemic signs and symptoms.
   - **d.** Systemic signs and symptoms related to pregnancy.
2. *Physical examination* should include a complete evaluation with specific emphasis upon the genitalia after hemodynamic stability has been assured.
   - **a.** Complete pelvic examination to exclude trauma, discharge, excoriation, masses, tenderness, or other pathology.
   - **b.** Survey to evaluate for endocrine dysfunction.
   - **c.** Abdominal examination.
3. *Diagnostic work-up*.
   - **a.** Laboratory.
     - **(1)** Cultures, Gram's stain, and saline and KOH preparation of any vaginal discharge. *Neisseria gonorrhoeae* and *Chlamydia trachomatis* should be specifically sought. Pap smear if indicated.
     - **(2)** CBC, ESR, endocrine assessment, bleeding screen, as appropriate.

Table 27-1. Vaginal Bleeding: Etiologic Considerations

Condition	Diagnostic Findings	Comments
Endocrine		
Uterine dysfunction	Irregular menses, flow frequent, heavy, prolonged	Anovulatory cycle; early menstrual pattern
Pregnancy complications		
Abortion-threatened	First trimester; enlarged nontender uterus, closed cervix	If os open, inevitable abortion; if closed, 30–40% chance of carrying pregnancy
Abortion-incomplete	First trimester bleeding, cramps, cervical dilation; enlarged, tender uterus; os open; Hct	Products of conception may be visible; profuse bleeding
Abortion-complete	First trimester complete expulsion products conception; small uterus; os open	Hct
Ectopic pregnancy	Missed menses; pelvic pain, rebound, adnexal mass; hypotension; Hct	Ultrasound, culdocentesis; positive pregnancy test; life-threatening
Placenta previa	Third trimester; painless, profuse bleeding	Ultrasound
Abruptio placentae	Third trimester; abdominal pain, tender uterus; concealed bleeding	Ultrasound; follows blunt trauma
Polycystic ovary	Enlarged ovary	Ultrasound
Adrenal disorder	Irregular menses, associated findings	Endocrine evaluation
Thyroid disease	Irregular menses, associated findings	Thyroid functions
Diabetes mellitus	Irregular menses, associated findings	Evaluation glucose metabolism
Obesity or weight loss	Irregular menses, recent change weight	Dietary, psychiatric changes
Physiologic	Blood tinged or bloody, discharge in newborn during first 5–10 days	Withdrawal from maternal estrogens
Trauma		
Foreign body	Foul smelling discharge	Peak is 5–9 years (cotton, tissues, etc.); older women (tampon, IUD, etc.)
Laceration	Signs of trauma	Due to trauma, exercise, intercourse, molestation, abuse

Inflammation/Infection		
Vulvovaginitis	Discharge, inflamed introitus, dysuria	Culture, saline and KOH prep
Pelvic inflammatory disease	Abdominal, pelvic tenderness, fever, chills; toxic	Elevated CBC and ESR, culture, Gram's stain
Enterobius vermicularis	Nighttime rectal pruritus; excoriation	"Scotch tape" test; common prepubertal
Intrauterine device	Excessive cramping, bleeding	
Intoxication		
Birth control pills	Irregular intake, overdose	Inadequate estrogens
Anticoagulants	Bleeding site elsewhere	Bleeding screen
Deficiency		
Bleeding diathesis	Bleeding site elsewhere	Bleeding screen
Iron deficiency anemia	Impaired production or blood loss	Anemia evaluation
Idiopathic thrombocytopenia purpura	Bleeding site elsewhere	Bleeding screen
Neoplasm		
Tumors, polyps, fibroid, leiomyoma	Physical exam reveals mass; spotting or bleeding	Unusual; may occur in children exposed to diethylstilbestrol (DES) in utero: Pap smear

(3) Pregnancy test. About 14 days before the next expected menstruation, ovulation is triggered by a surge of luteinizing hormone (LH). Nine days later (1 or 2 days after implantation), human chorionic gonadotropin (HCG) becomes detectable. HCG maintains the corpus luteum of pregnancy, supporting the excretion of estrogen and progesterone. HCG initially increases every 2 days so that by the expected day of menstruation, the HCG level is 50 mIU/ml, 2 days later 100 mIU/ml, and so on. By the sixth week of gestation (2 weeks after the first missed period) the level is 3,000 mIU/ml, peaking at 8–12 weeks with levels of 20,000–100,000 mIU/ml, and declining during the third trimester.
   (a) Latex agglutination-inhibition is useful 45 days after the last menstrual period for the diagnosis of routine pregnancies.
   (b) Radioimmunoassay (RIA) can detect pregnancy 8–13 days after conception.
   (c) Monoclonal antibody agglutination correlates well with RIA and is cheaper and easier to perform.
(4) Pathological examination as indicated.
(5) Bleeding screening (PT, PTT, bleeding time, platelets).

b. Radiologic examination should include an ultrasound, which may be useful to confirm an intrauterine pregnancy and identify pelvic pathology.

Alert: Hemodynamic stability should be assessed while evaluating contributing conditions.

Bibliography

Emans SJH and Goldstein DP: *Pediatric and Adolescent Gynecology* (2d ed.). Boston: Little Brown, 1982.

Farrell RG (ed.): *Ob-Gyn Emergencies: The First 60 Minutes*. Rockville: Aspen Pub, 1988.

Litt I: Menstrual problems during adolescence. Pediatr Rev 7:203, 1983.

28 Vaginal Discharge

Vaginal discharge is common in prepubertal and pubescent females. The discharge reflects the underlying cause and the age of the patient (Table 28-1).

Etiologic Considerations

Prepubertal girls develop discharge because of the relatively thin mucosa, the close proximity to the rectum, and the alkaline pH of vaginal secretions. Additional contributing factors include poor personal hygiene, irritation from bubble bath or sand, foreign bodies, and infection (*Chlamydia trachomatis, Neisseria gonorrhoeae, Trichomonas vaginalis*, group A streptococcus, *Shigella* species, and *Yersinia*, the first three often being associated with sexual abuse).

A thick, mucoid discharge is not uncommon in the newborn, reflecting estrogen withdrawal. The discharge may be blood tinged or bloody and resolves by 10 days.

Pubescent females have discharge due to those entities causing problems in younger children as well as the changing hormone and pH balance, greater sexual activity, and enhanced exposure.

Also see Chap. 27.

Table 28-1. Vaginal Discharge: Etiologic Considerations

Condition	Diagnostic Findings	Comments
Infection		
Candida albicans	Discharge: thick, white, cheeselike; dysuria; hyphae on KOH prep	Nystatin, miconidazole
Neisseria gonorrhoeae	Discharge: purulent or minimal; PID; dysuria; Gram's stain and culture	Penicillin, amoxicillin
Chlamydia trachomatis	Discharge: purulent; dysuria	Doxycycline
Trichomonas vaginalis	Discharge: thin, frothy, yellow-green, malodorous; dysuria; pruritus, abdominal pain; saline prep: motile trichomonads	Metronidazole
Gardnerella vaginalis	Discharge: gray/clear, fishy smell, "clue" cells; pruritus	Metronidazole
Herpes simplex, type 2	Group vesicles with variable discharge; dysuria, pruritus	Acyclovir
Trauma		
Foreign body	Discharge: foul smelling; sand, tampon, etc.	Peak in 5–9-year-olds
Irritation, maceration	Variable discharge; bubble bath, poor hygiene, chemical douche, IUD, deodorant, contraceptive spray, etc.	

Diagnostic Approach

1. *History* should focus on gynecologic problems.
   a. Menstrual and sexual history including exposures, recurrence, previous treatment. Exclude possibility of trauma or abuse, in utero DES exposure, any foreign bodies.
   b. Other systemic findings including evidence of toxicity or abdominal tenderness consistent with pelvic inflammatory disease (PID).
2. *Physical examination* should concentrate on the genitalia and abdomen. Pelvic examination to determine the nature of the discharge and any pelvic or abdominal tenderness, rebound, or guarding. Special attention should be given to defining bruises, lacerations, or scrapes. Tremendous care must be exercised in performing a pelvic examination in the young girl. This must be done with patience, clear explanations, and sensitivity, usually in the mother's presence.
3. *Diagnostic work-up*.
   a. Laboratory evaluation should include cultures, Gram's stain, and saline and KOH preparation of vaginal discharge.
   b. Therapeutic trial, removal of potential irritants or removal of foreign body.

   Alert: Sexual activity should be considered in children who have an infectious origin for any discharge.

Bibliography

Abramowicz M: Treatment of sexually transmitted diseases. Med Litt Drugs Ther 30:5, 1988.

Golden N, Cohen H, Gennari G, et al.: The use of pelvic ultrasonography in the evaluation of adolescents with pelvic inflammatory disease. Am J Dis Child 141:1235, 1987.

Sanders LJ, Harrson HR, and Washington AE: Treatment of sexually transmitted chlamydial infections. JAMA 255:1750, 1986.

X

Hematologic Problems

29 Anemia

Children with a red cell volume or hemoglobin concentration below the third percentile for the patient's age group are anemic. In general, a hemoglobin level below 11 gm/dl is consistent with anemia, although there is marked age-specific variability (see Figure 29-1). Anemia is commonly a manifestation of primary disease or nutritional deficiency.

Dehydration may decrease the plasma volume, artificially elevating the hemoglobin while congestive heart failure may cause a dilutional effect. During rapid acute blood loss, initial hemotocrits may show little decrease because of the period of equilibrium. Serial monitoring is necessary.

(See also p. 238.)

Etiologic Considerations

1. Anemia is caused by *inadequate erythropoiesis* due to impaired red cell production, maturation, or release from the bone marrow. Iron deficiency anemia is by far the most common cause.
   a. Nutritional iron deficiency is the most common cause of anemia in children between 6 months and 2 years of age. Typically, it results from excessive cow's milk intake and inadequate consumption of iron-rich foods as the child outgrows newborn iron stores. Iron deficiency anemia in children over 2 years of age should be investigated for the possibility of chronic blood loss. Children may be irritable and have learning problems and delayed motor development. Severe deficiency may lead to a protein losing enteropathy with blood in the stools.
   b. Physiologic anemia of infancy. The rapid increase in blood volume leads to a relative anemia with the hemoglobin values typically being 10.5 gm/dl at 2 months and 11 gm/dl at 3 months of age. Prematures often have an even further exaggeration of anemia, falling in the normal preterm infant to as low as 8 gm/dl at 2–3 months of age.
   c. Copper, folate, B_{12}, or B_6 deficiency. Associated with impaired maturation of bone marrow red cell precursors.
   d. Thalassemia syndromes, lead poisoning, sideroblastic anemia, and pyridoxine deficiency are due to impaired hemoglobin production. Thalassemia also has associated intramedullary hemolysis.
   e. Chronic disease or inflammation: renal disease, hypopituitarism, and hypothyroidism impair production.
   f. Malignancy and storage disease cause marrow replacement and infiltration.
   g. Fanconi's anemia, Blackfan-Diamond anemia, transient erythroblastopenia of childhood (TEC), aplastic anemia (drugs, radiation, infection, malignancy, hepatitis, idiopathic).
2. *Hemolytic destruction or sequestration* of circulating red cells. Cells normally have a life span of 100–120 days; hemolysis due to a variety of conditions may dramatically shorten this period, leading to anemia.
   a. Hemoglobinopathies include sickle cell disorders, thalassemia, hemoglobin variants, and persistence of fetal hemoglobin causing hemolysis and often splenic sequestration.

Figure 29-1. Evaluation of anemia. (Reproduced by permission from Barkin RM and Rosen P: *Emergency Pediatrics: A Guide to Ambulatory Care* (3rd ed.). St. Louis: C. V. Mosby Co., 1990.)

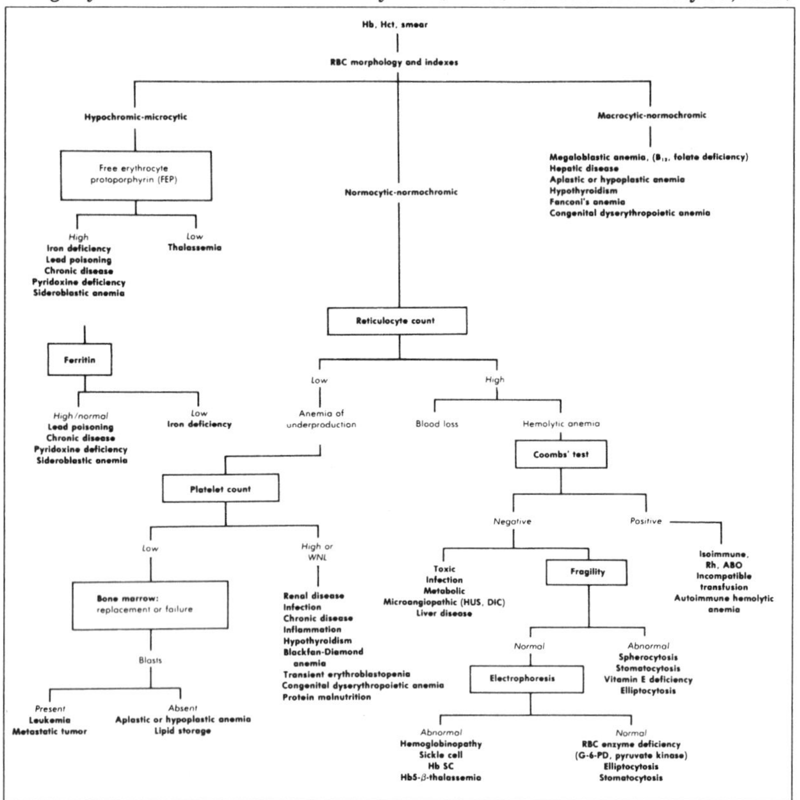

  - **b.** Erythrocyte membrane defects may be associated with abnormal osmotic fragility, elliptocytosis, and enzymatic defects producing nondeformable cells.
  - **c.** Extracorpuscular damage secondary to microangiopathic hemolytic anemia, prosthetic heart valve, hemangioma, cardiac defect, hemolytic uremic syndrome (HUS). It may also be primary due to an autoimmune hemolytic anemia (idiopathic).
  - **d.** Portal hypertension produces splenic sequestration.

3. *Blood loss*, either of an acute or chronic nature. Trauma, surgery, bleeding disorder, and peptic ulcer disease are but a few underlying conditions. The degree of anemia is affected by the rapidity of the blood loss. With chronic blood loss, there may be a complicating iron deficiency anemia.

Diagnostic Approach

1. *History* must include specific factors that help define the underlying condition.
   - **a.** Age, sex, ethnic background, and diet.
   - **b.** Duration and nature of symptoms. Pallor, fatigue, dizziness, amenorrhea, and so on. These reflect the severity of the anemia, rapidity of onset, and underlying etiology.
     - **(1)** With rapid onset of anemia, headache, dizziness, postural hypotension, tachycardia, and high-output cardiac failure may be present.

(2) Insidious onset is typically associated with pallor, fatigue, and decreased exercise tolerance.

c. Chronic illness and infection, bleeding, drugs, and pica.

d. Family history of anemia, jaundice, gallbladder disease, splenomegaly, or splenectomy. Ancestry may be suggestive of sickle cell disease, thalassemia, or G6PD deficiency.

e. Response to previous therapy, such as iron.

f. Menstrual history regarding regularity, frequency, and amount (e.g., number of pads).

2. *Physical examination.*

a. Vital signs and any evidence of cardiovascular instability, delayed capillary refill, orthostatic changes, evidence of pallor, petechiae, purpura, and ecchymoses.

b. Lymphadenopathy, blood in stool, and signs associated with complications (e.g., hypoxia, splenomegaly, congestive heart failure) and any underlying conditions.

3. *Diagnostic work-up* should be done systematically using the protocol outlined in Figure 29-1. Initially, develop potential diagnostic considerations on the basis of the history, physical, and blood count and review the smear and indices to make sure they are consistent. Then either a therapeutic trial or further diagnostic evaluation is indicated.

a. Laboratory studies should include:

(1) Complete blood count (hemoglobin, hematocrit, and RBC indexes), blood smear, and reticulocyte count. Indices are particularly useful in defining the differential considerations. Serial hematocrits may be required in monitoring blood loss.

(2) Anemia with microcytosis suggests iron deficiency. Determine the free-erythrocyte protoporphyrin (FEP) or serum ferritin. An FEP greater than 2.8 μg/g of Hgb and a serum ferritin of less than 10 ng/ml are typical of iron deficiency. Iron saturation (serum iron/total iron-binding capacity × 100) of less than 20% is also indicative of iron deficiency but is subject to greater error because of diurnal and acute diet-related fluctuations in serum iron. An FEP of greater than 17.5 μg/g of Hgb strongly suggests lead poisoning.

(3) Stool for occult blood.

(4) Studies specific for potential etiology, including Coombs test, serum folate or B_{12} levels, evidence of hemolysis (bilirubin, fecal/urinary urobilinogen excretion, and serum haptoglobin), intracorpuscular defect screening for fragility, screening tests for infection, bilirubin, hemoglobin electrophoresis, and so on.

Other specific studies may include fibrinogen, fibrin split products (FSP), ANA, and rheumatoid factor.

(5) Bone marrow biopsy may be appropriate in the unresponsive and undiagnosed patient who is refractory to normal therapy and for whom the consideration of systemic disease is high.

b. Therapeutic trial in the patient with hypochromic microcytic anemia may be appropriate in healthy children. A trial of elemental iron 5 mg/kg/24 hr q 8 hr PO may be therapeutic using ferrous sulfate (Fer-in-Sol) 75 mg (15 mg elemental iron)/0.6 ml dropper. The reticulocyte count should increase within 3–5 days and the hemoglobin rises after about one week. Therapy is continued for 2 months.

Alert: Iron deficiency is the most common underlying condition but all children need to be evaluated for instability and then for potential contributing conditions.

Bibliography

Dallman P, Yip R, and Johnson C: Prevalence and causes of anemia in the United States, 1976–1980. Am J Clin Nutr 39:437, 1985.

Oski FA and Stockman JA III: Anemia due to inadequate iron stores or poor iron utilization. Pediatr Clin North Am 27:237, 1980.

30 Bleeding

Bleeding may occur in children due to injury as well as a variety of congenital or acquired conditions. It is essential to distinguish normal bleeding following trauma from abnormal bleeding that occurs with minimal or no injury.

Etiologic Considerations

Patterns of bleeding differ, reflecting the type of defect and the nature and location of the injury. Bleeding may reflect a primary abnormality in platelets or capillary function due to, for example, liver dysfunction, uremia, or aspirin ingestion, or it may reflect a deficiency in specific hemostatic factors (Table 30-1).

Diagnostic Approach

1. *Historical* focus must determine the nature of the bleeding, as delineated above.
   a. A history of bleeding problems through prior experience with procedures, such as circumcision, lacerations, tooth extraction, or menstruation, that typically cause transient bleeding.
   b. A thorough family history is essential.
2. *Physical findings* must determine the nature of the bleeding and potential hemodynamic complications.
   a. The site, extent, and nature of bleeding after assessment of vital signs including orthostatics to ensure that there is no significant blood loss.
   b. Underlying tissue should be evaluated to assure no involvement. If bruises or bleeding are unexplained or inconsistent with the history, additional evaluation for child abuse should be considered.

Table 30-1. Bleeding: Etiologic Considerations

	Platelet/Capillary Defect	Coagulation Factor Defect
Preceding injury		
None (spontaneous)	Small, diffuse bleeding of mucous membranes	Major musculoskeletal or CNS bleeding
Superficial cut	Profuse, prolonged	Minimal
Deep cut	Immediate, good response to pressure	Delayed; poor response to pressure
Joint trauma	Hemarthrosis uncommon	Hemarthrosis common
Petechiae	Common	Rare
Diagnostic work-up	Prolonged BT, abnormal platelets	Prolonged PTT, PT

3. *Diagnostic work-up* is required to delineate specific components of a screening for bleeding in addition to evaluating the specific injury as required. Findings are outlined as found in a variety of specific conditions (Table 30-2).

   Laboratory.

   a. CBC, peripheral blood smear, and platelet count.
   b. Bleeding time (BT).
   c. Partial thromboplastin time (PTT), prothrombin time (PT), and thrombin time (TT).
   d. Fibrinogen.
   e. Specific factor assays.
   f. Platelet-function studies.

   Alert: Recurrent bleeding requires evaluation, while that following injury requires a systematic approach to trauma.

Bibliography

Buchanan G: Hemophilia. Pediatr Clin North Am 27:309, 1980.

Montgomery RR and Hathaway WF: Acute bleeding emergencies. Pediatr Clin North Am 27:327, 1980.

Table 30-2. Screening of the Bleeding Patient

	Screening Tests					
Condition	Platelet Count	BT	PTT	PT	TT	Comments
Normal (WNL) (varies with lab)	150–400,000/ml	4–9 min	25–35 sec	12–13 sec	8–10 sec	Fibrinogen 190–400 mg/dl
Hereditary Disorders						
Hemophilia						
Factor VIII (Classic: A)	WNL	WNL	↑	WNL	WNL	Factor assay
Factor IX (Christmas: B)	WNL	WNL	↑	WNL	WNL	Factor assay
Factor XI	WNL	WNL	↑	WNL	WNL	Factor assay
Factor XII	WNL	WNL	↑	WNL	WNL	Factor assay
Factor II, V, X	WNL	WNL	↑	↑	WNL	Factor assay
Factor VII	WNL	WNL	WNL	↑	WNL	Factor assay
von Willebrand's (many variants)	WNL	↑	↑	WNL	WNL	VIII antigen, VIII cofactor, ristocetin cofactor
Platelet dysfunction	WNL/↓	↑	WNL	WNL	WNL	Platelet aggregation studies
Acquired Disorders						
Disseminated intravascular coagulation	↓	↑	↑	↑	↑	↓ fibrinogen, ↑ fibrin spilt products
Idiopathic thrombocytopenic purpura	↓	↑	WNL	WNL	WNL	
Henoch-Schönlein purpura	WNL	WNL	WNL	WNL	WNL	
Liver failure (severe)	WNL/↓	WNL/↑	↑	↑	WNL/↑	↓ fibrinogen, ↑ fibrin split products

Uremia (p. 660)	WNL/↓	↑	WNL	WNL	WNL/↑	Secondary to hepatic dysfunction or protein loss
Anticoagulants						
Heparin	WNL	WNL	↑	WNL/↑	↑ ↑	Also lupus-like and inactivating anticoagulant
Coumadin	WNL	WNL	WNL/↑	↑	WNL	
Aspirin	WNL	↑	WNL	WNL	WNL	

(Reproduced by permission from Barkin RM and Rosen P: *Emergency Pediatrics: A Guide to Ambulatory Care* (3rd ed.). St. Louis: C.V. Mosby Co., 1990.)

XI Metabolic and Endocrine Problems

31 Hypoglycemia

Hypoglycemia is a reflection of the balance between glucose production and peripheral glucose utilization. Hypoglycemia may result from inadequate endogenous glucose substrate (alanine, lactate, and glycerol), dysfunctional glucose synthesis or storage, or enhanced utilization (hormonal regulation).

Blood glucose concentrations diagnostic of hypoglycemia are age dependent. A blood glucose of less than 40 mg/dl in the child, 30 mg/dl in the full-term infant, and 20 mg/dl in the preterm infant is considered abnormal.

Etiologic Considerations

Newborns experience transient hypoglycemia, often associated with perinatal complications due to excessive insulin secretion including maternal diabetes or erythroblastosis. Beyond the first day of life, and often associated with hypoxia and intrauterine growth retardation, is a more prolonged hypoglycemia due to inadequate glycogen stores. Congenital abnormalities of the central nervous system or heart may cause hypoglycemia; sepsis and hypocalcemia may develop.

During *infancy*, inborn errors of carbohydrate and glycogen storage, amino acid and organic acid metabolism, as well as endocrine abnormalities, cause hypoglycemia during the first year of life. Hypoglycemia typically occurs shortly after the ingestion of protein in patients with idiopathic leucine sensitivity and defects in amino acid and organic acid metabolism. Ingestion of lactose may stimulate hypoglycemia associated with galactosemia, while sucrose ingestion may produce hypoglycemia in the presence of hereditary fructose intolerance.

Beyond one year of life, fasting hypoglycemia may result from ketotic hypoglycemia or, less commonly, hormonal deficiencies, hyperinsulinism, glycogen storage disease, or fructose 1,6-diphosphatase (FDPase) deficiency. Preschool and elementary school children may be symptomatic following prolonged fasting, exacerbating the physiologic response to starvation. Poisons or toxins may be contributory in other patients (Table 31-1).

Inborn Errors of Metabolism

These disorders may be associated with metabolic acidosis, ketonemia, or hepatomegaly (Chap. 25). Distinctions that may be useful include:

1. *Nonketotic* hypoglycemia with hepatomegaly suggests 3-hydroxy-3 methylglutaric aciduria, glutaric aciduria type II, systemic carnitine deficiency or carnitine palmitoyl transferase deficiency.
2. *Ketotic* hypoglycemia usually has an onset of 1½–5 years of age and is resolved by 9 or 10 years of age. Hypopituitarism and ACTH responsiveness should be considered.
3. *Nonglucose reducing substances* in the urine suggest galactosemia and hereditary fructose intolerance.
4. *Hyperammonemia* is present in children with organic acid and amino acid metabolism defects.
5. *Hyperinsulinemia* commonly has no ketonuria or metabolic acidosis.

Table 31-1. Hypoglycemia: Etiologic Considerations

	Inborn Error of metabolism (carbohydrate/ amino acid)	Hormonal deficiency	Hyperinsulinism
History			
Hypoglycemia			
Fasting	Common* (many hrs)	Common (few hrs)	Common (few hrs)
After lactose	Galactosemia	No	No
After sucrose	Hereditary fructose intolerance	No	No
After protein	Amino acid, organic acid	No	No
Family history	Common	Variable	Variable
Physical			
Hepatomegaly	Common	No	No
Failure to thrive	Common	Variable	Variable
Laboratory			
Ketosis	Common**	Variable	No
Acidosis	Common	No	No
Nonglucose urine reducing substance	Galactosemia, hereditary fructose intolerance		
Hyperammonemia	Amino acid, organic acid		
Liver function abnormality	Common	No	No

*Glycogen storage disease. Fructose-1, 6-diphosphatase deficiency.
**If no ketosis, consider 3-hydroxy-3-methylglutaric aciduria, glutaric aciduria type II, systemic carnitine deficiency, and carnitine palmitoyl transferase deficiency.

Carbohydrate enzyme defects result from deficiencies of hepatic glucose formation and release (Chap. 25).

1. *Glycogen storage disease* may cause growth retardation, cherubic features, protuberant abdomen, large smooth liver, enlarged kidney, initial normal intelligence, fasting hypoglycemia after only a few hours, ketosis, lactic acidemia, hyperlipidemia, hyperuricemia, bleeding diathesis.
2. *Galactosemia* causes failure to thrive (FTT), jaundice, vomiting, susceptibility to infection, hepatomegaly, edema, ascites, tendency to bleed, cataracts, proteinuria, aminoaciduria, and galactosuria. May progress to develop mental retardation, progressive liver disease, and death.
3. *Hereditary fructose intolerance* with fructose ingestion produces vomiting, profound hypoglycemia, and convulsions. May progress to failure to thrive, vomiting, jaundice, hepatosplenomegaly, hemorrhage, abnormal liver function, fructosuria, defect in proximal renal tubular function, hepatic failure, and death.
4. *FDPase deficiency* produces episodic hyperventilation, fasting hypoglycemia, lactic acidosis, ketosis, hyperuricemia, and hepatomegaly.

Amino acid and organic acid metabolic defects may begin in neonatal period. Improves with cessation of protein feeding.

Hyperinsulism

1. *Beta cell abnormalities:* islet cell adenoma, focal adenomatosis, beta-cell hyperplasia.
2. *Leucine sensitivity* usually does not cause symptoms until 1–6 months of age.
3. *Beckwith-Wiedemann syndrome:* omphalocele, macroglossia, gigantism, and hypoglycemia in 3–50% of infants secondary to beta cell hyperplasia. May also have hemihypertrophy as well as increased incidence of adrenal, liver, kidney (Wilm's) tumors.
4. *Nesidioblastosis* has beta cells throughout acinar tissue and neoformation of islet cells budding off from ductile elements. This is the most common cause of hyperinsulinism in the first year of life and may be associated with hypoglycemia later.
5. Pancreatic islet cell *adenoma* is uncommon. Usually onset is after 4 years of age.

Hormone Deficiency

1. *Hypopituitarism* is congenital due to hypothalamic abnormality, aplasia of the anterior pituitary. May have midline defects, including hypertelorism, abnormality of the frontal growth hormone deficiency.
2. *Cortisol deficiency* due to Addison's disease, congenital adrenal hyperplasia, ACTH deficiency, ACTH unresponsiveness.

Ketotic Hypoglycemia

This is the most common cause of hypoglycemia after 1 year of age. Ketonuria, hypoglycemia, and central nervous symptoms have a peak incidence at 2 years of age. It may be an exaggeration of the starvation state.

Poison or Toxin

Salicylates.
Alcohol.
Oral hypoglycemic agents.
Insulin.
Beta-adrenergic agents (e.g., propranolol).

Miscellaneous

Liver disease due to hepatitis or cirrhosis.
Malnutrition presenting as kwashiorkor, starvation, or malabsorption.

Diagnostic Approach

1. *Historically*, information should focus on the pattern of evolution of the symptomatic hypoglycemia.
   a. Age of onset of hypoglycemia and the nature of episodes should be explored with particular reference to the frequency of clinical signs and symptoms such as dizziness, vomiting, failure to thrive, change in mental status, irritability, loss of consciousness, and seizures; response to glucose (or glucagon) administration; and the temporal relationship to food intake.
   b. Perinatal problems and a family history of seizures, hypoglycemia, failure to thrive, and early death should be excluded. If other family members have a history of hypoglycemia, the pattern of episodes should be explored.
   c. Family history of abnormal glucose metabolism such as diabetes or hypoglycemia.
   d. Recent medication ingestion.
2. *Physical examination* should focus on hemodynamic stability.
   a. Stability of airway, ventilation, and circulation should be evaluated.
   b. Mental status should be assessed, as should evidence of liver failure or enlargement. Specific sequelae of individual diseases should also be sought.

3. *Diagnostic work-up* should determine the severity of the hypoglycemia.

a. Laboratory evaluation should include immediate data.

(1) Chemistry: serial serum glucose, ketone, and pH. Bedside measurements of glucose may be adequate. A glucose tolerance test may be valuable. Others would measure glucose during prolonged dieting. Specific specialized tests such as organic and amino acid determinations, toxicology screens, and liver function analyses are commonly required.

(2) Specific entities such as response to fasting, exposure to leucine, and so on.

b. Therapeutic trials should initially focus on administration of parenteral glucose, monitoring for a response. Specific attention may also be addressed to excluding diagnostic considerations.

Alert: Hypoglycemia is a common cause of altered mental status and often requires empirical treatment with parenteral glucose.

Bibliography

Cornblath M: Hypoglycemia in infancy and childhood. Pediatr Ann 10:356, 1981.

LaFranchi S: Hypoglycemia of infancy and childhood. Pediatr Clin North Am 34:961, 1987.

Phillip M, Bashan N, Smith CPH, et al.: An algorithm approach to diagnosis of hypoglycemia. J Pediatr 110:287, 1987.

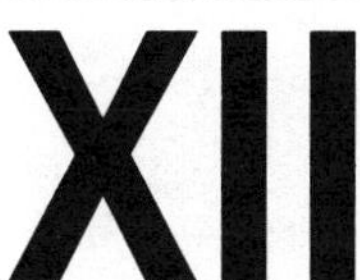

XII Neurologic Problems

32 Altered Mental Status

Children may experience alteration in mental status from a variety of conditions, the relative alteration from normal being a continuum (Table 32-1). Children may be *confused* with a reduced awareness of environment and responsiveness or be *delusional*, usually accompanied by agitation and impaired responsiveness. Progression to *stupor* occurs when the child can be awakened only with repeated, vigorous stimuli; ultimately the unresponsiveness of coma may evolve.

Physiologically, there is usually hypoxia or other metabolic deficit such as hypoglycemia, direct tissue injury, or increased intracranial pressure with displacement from an enlargement of one of the cranial cavity components: brain tissue, cerebral spinal fluid, and blood.

Etiologic Considerations

In considering potential etiologies, the underlying process and anatomical location assist in defining the contributing condition. Mnemonics have been used extensively in simplifying the differential of the most common etiologies. Two systems (I SPOUT A VEIN and AEIOU TIPS) that have been suggested are:

Insulin	**A**lcohol
Shock (poor perfusion)	**E**ncephalopathy/encephalitis/electrolytes-metabolic
Psychogenic	**I**nsulin/intussusception
Overdose	**O**verdose
Uremia-metabolic	**U**remia-metabolic
Trauma	**T**rauma
Alcohol	**I**nfection
	Psychiatric
Vascular	**S**eizure
Encephalopathy	
Infection	
Neoplasm	

Supratentorial lesions have findings suggestive of focal hemispheric pathology that progress from a rostal to a caudal direction. Pupillary reactions are usually depressed and motor signs are asymmetrical. *Infratentorial* pathology is associated with brainstem dysfunction; evolution is not orderly. Respiratory patterns are abnormal and cranial nerve palsies are common.

Metabolic abnormalities are usually diffuse, having an impact on mental status before symmetrical motor findings develop. Pupillary reactions are preserved and seizures are common.

Diagnostic Approach

1. *Historically*, a complete description of the progression of mental status alteration is essential.
   a. Level of responsiveness, onset, progression, recurrence.

Table 32-1. Altered Mental Status: Etiologic Considerations

Condition	Diagnostic Findings	Comments
Infection		
Meningitis	Fever, headache, lethargy, irritability, rare focal findings; CSF: Increased WBC and protein, decreased glucose	Concurrent infection; bacterial or viral
Encephalitis	Fever, headache, tremor, ataxia, cranial nerve VI palsy, irritable, lethargic; rare focal findings; CSF: increased WBC and protein; normal glucose	Viral: measles, mumps, rubella, EB virus (infectious mono); Bacterial: pertussis, immunization
Subdural empyema/ intracranial abscess	Fever, headache, focal findings, increased intracranial pressure; CSF: increased WBC, protein, and pressure, culture negative; CT scan; subdural tap	Empyema may follow trauma, meningitis; abscess may be extension otitis, mastoiditis
Trauma		
Cerebral concussion	Dizziness, vomiting, headache, amnesia, transient blindness; no focal findings; CT scan	Follows trauma; rule out mass lesion
Subdural hematoma	Altered mentation after trauma; headache, focal findings; CT scan	Rapid progression; rare delay
Epidural hematoma	Often a period of lucidity, lapsing into stupor or coma; focal findings; CT scan	Delayed onset
Drowning	No focal findings; CT variable	Reflects hypoxia
Heat stroke	Febrile (> 40°C), headache, confusion, acidosis; CSF, CT: normal	History exposure
Endocrine/Metabolic		
Hypoglycemia (Chap. 31)	Sweating, pallor, tachycardia, tremor, seizures	< 40 mg/dl in child; > 30 mg/dl newborn; empirical response to glucose
Diabetic ketoacidosis	Kussmaul's breathing, orthostatic; polydipsia, polyuria; acidosis; no focal findings; electrolytes, ABG normal	Compliance or intercurrent illness
Hypo-/hypernatremia	Dehydration, edema, seizure; no focal findings	Multiple etiologies; adrenal failure, Ca^{++}, Mg^{++}, etc.

Uremia/renal failure	Decreased urine output, edema, lethargy; CHF, dysrhythmia, hypertension; no focal findings; BUN, creatinine, electrolytes abnormal	Multiple etiologies: prerenal, renal, obstructive
Reye's syndrome	Lethargy, stupor, agitation, hepatic dysfunction; increased intracranial pressure; no focal findings; liver functions abnormal; LP normal; ammonia elevated	Follows URI with vomiting; multiple etiologies
Inborn errors of metabolism (Chap. 25)	Variable presentation	Multiple types, etiologies
Intoxication		
Sedatives/hypnotics/narcotics	Progressive deterioration mentation; miotic (narcotic); hypotension; no focal findings	Empirical response to naloxone (Narcan)
Ethanol	Lethargy, ataxia, slurred speech; visual hallucinations, poor coordination; seizure; no focal findings; ethanol level	Associated level depends upon chronicity
Carbon monoxide	Headache, dizziness, vomiting, progressive deterioration; no focal findings; carboxyhemoglobin level	Empirical response to oxygen
Vascular		
Shock (Chap. 3)	Hypotension, multiple organ failure	Inadequate perfusion, hypoxia
Hypertensive encephalopathy (Chap. 12)	Escalating blood pressure; headache, vomiting, hemiparesis; CT scan	Multiple etiologies; response to lower BP
Cerebral vascular accident/stroke	Rapid onset; focal findings, hemiplegia, papilledema, proptosis, conjunctival hemorrhage, ophthalmoplegia (cavernous sinus thrombosis)	Rare in children; underlying disease: cyanotic heart disease, sickle cell, endocarditis, trauma
Other		
Epilepsy	Postictal period following seizure; may be focal (Todd's paralysis); EEG	Multiple etiologies
Hysteria	Inconsistent, recurrent findings	
Neoplasm	Variable findings; CT scan	

b. Family history of impaired responsiveness, cerebral vascular accident, stroke, cyanotic heart disease, sickle cell disease, diabetes mellitus, hypoglycemia, inborn errors of metabolism.
c. Trauma, recent illness, intoxication, exposure to carbon monoxide, lead, excessive heat, psychiatric illness, or drowning.

2. *Physical examination* in the child with impaired mental status should assist in defining the nature of the injury as well as possible contributing conditions.

Determine the patient's respiratory, cardiovascular, and neurological stability during the initial evaluation and then proceed to a thorough neurological examination, which should assess cranial nerves; motor, sensory, and cerebellar function; and mental status.

a. *Respiratory* patterns should be assessed to determine the level of the rostro-caudal cerebral pathology.
   (1) Hyperventilation.
      (a) Compensation for metabolic acidosis (methanol, uremia, diabetes, drug ingestion).
      (b) Primary respiratory alkalosis (hepatic coma, pulmonary disease, psychogenic).
      (c) Central neurogenic hyperventilation due to midbrain dysfunction.
      (d) Compensation for hypoxia.
   (2) Hypoventilation.
      (a) Compensation for metabolic alkalosis (ingestion or loss of acid through GI or GU tract).
      (b) Respiratory acidosis (pulmonary, CNS, or neuromuscular disease).
   (3) Cheynes-Stokes respiration with periods of hyperpnea followed by hyperpnoia.
      Bilateral hemisphere dysfunction with intact brain stem. May also be due to metabolic abnormality or incipient temporal lobe herniation.
b. *Position* may reflect posturing.
   (1) Decorticate posturing occurs when the arms are flexed and abducted and the legs extended. Corticospinal tract lesion within or near the cerebral hemisphere.
   (2) Decerebrate posturing has the arms extended and internally rotated against the chest with the legs extended.
      (a) Midbrain to midpons lesions.
      (b) Metabolic abnormality (hypoxia, hypoglycemia).
      (c) Bilateral hemispheric lesion.
c. *Pupils*.
   (1) Pinpoint (1–2 mm) and fixed.
      (a) Pontine lesion.
      (b) Metabolic abnormality or intoxication (narcotic).
   (2) Small (2–3 mm) and reactive.
      (a) Medullary lesion.
      (b) Metabolic abnormality.
   (3) Dilated and fixed.
      (a) Bilateral: irreversible brain damage, anticholinergic drugs, barbiturates, hypothermia, seizures.
      (b) Unilateral: rapidly expanding lesion on ipsilateral side (subdural hematoma, tumor), tentorial herniation, lesion of cranial nerve III, anticholinergic eye drops, seizures.
   (4) Dilated and reactive.
      (a) Postictal.
      (b) Anticholinergic drugs.
d. *Eye movement*.
   (1) Occulocephalic reflex (doll's eye): with the eyes held open, the head is quickly turned from side to side. Normally, the eyes will move in the direction opposite to which the head is turned, as if gazing ahead in the initial position. Comatose patient with midbrain or pons lesion will have random movement. Cervical spine must be uninjured to test.
   (2) Oculovestibular reflex with caloric stimulation: with the head elevated 30 degrees, up to 200 ml (adult) ice water injected into the ear canal via a catheter will

normally result in conjugate deviation of the eyes to the irrigated ear. Comatose patient with brainstem lesion will have no response.

- **(3)** Conjugate deviation.
  - **(a)** Cerebral lesion produces deviation toward destructive lesion and away from irritative pathology.
- **(4)** VI nerve palsy: eyes cannot move laterally.
  - **(a)** Increased intracranial pressure.
  - **(b)** Meningeal infection or irritation.
  - **(c)** Pontine lesion.
- **(5)** III nerve palsy: eyes point down and out.
  - **(a)** Tentorial herniation.
  - **(b)** Injury nerve-entrapment, lesion, compression.
  - **(c)** Brainstem lesions result in deviation away from destructive lesion. Lesions of the midbrain may produce setting sun sign with paralysis of upward gaze.
  - **(d)** Comatose patients with intact brain stem function normally have eyes directed straight ahead or minimally deviated.

3. *Diagnostic work-up* evaluation must follow a careful history, physical, and stabilization.

- **a.** Laboratory cvaluation should focus on potential etiologies.
  - **(1)** Chemistries: glucose, electrolytes. Consider liver functions, ammonia, BUN, and specialized tests as indicated.
  - **(2)** CBC to evaluate for infection.
  - **(3)** Arterial blood gas (or oximetry).
  - **(4)** Cultures of blood, etc. as appropriate.
  - **(5)** Lumbar punctures as indicated (Table 32-2).
  - **(6)** Urine and blood toxicology screen.
- **b.** Radiologically, a CT scan, often with contrast if nontraumatic condition considered.
- **c.** Therapeutic trial of oxygen, glucose, and naloxone is generally given during initial evaluation.

Alert: Ventilatory and hemodynamic stability must be achieved. Oxygen, glucose, and narcan may be given empirically and then diagnostic evaluation initiated.

Bibliography

American Academy of Pediatrics: *Report of the Committee on Infectious Diseases*, 21st ed. Elk Grove: American Academy of Pediatrics, 1988.

Berger MS, Pitts LH, Lovely M, et al.: Outcome from severe head injury in children and adolescents. J Neurosurg 62:194, 1985.

Dershewitz RA, Kaye BA, and Swisher CN: Treatment of children with post-traumatic loss of consciousness. Pediatrics 72:602, 1983.

Kennedy CR, Duffy SW, Smith R, et al.: Clinical predictors of outcome in encephalitis. Arch Dis Child 62:1156, 1987.

Nelson KB and Ellenberg JH: Prognosis in children with febrile seizures. Pediatrics 61:720, 1978.

Plum F and Posner JB: *The Diagnosis of Stupor and Coma* (3rd ed.). Philadelphia: FA Davis, 1980.

Table 32-2. Cerebrospinal Fluid Analysis

	Normal				
	Preterm	Term	>6 mo	Bacterial	Viral
Cell count (WBC/mm^3)*					
Mean	9	8	0	>500	<500
Range	0–25	0–22	0–4		
Predominant cell type	Lymph	Lymph	Lymph	80% PMN leukocyte	PMN leukocyte initially; lymphocyte later
Glucose (mg/dl)					
Mean	50	52	>40	<40	>40
Range	24–63	34–119			
Protein (mg/dl)					
Mean	115	90	<40	>100	<100
Range	65–150	20–170			
CSF/blood glucose (%)					
Mean	74	81	50	<40	>40
Range	55–150	44–248	40–60		
Gram's stain	Negative	Negative	Negative	Positive†	Negative
Bacterial culture	Negative	Negative	Negative	Positive‡	Negative

Modified from Sarff LD, Platt LH, and McCracken GH Jr: J Pediatr 88:473, 1976, and Portnoy JM and Olson LC: Pediatrics 75:484, 1985. (Reproduced by permission from Barkin RM and Rosen P: *Emergency Pediatrics: A Guide to Ambulatory Care* (3rd ed.). St. Louis: C. V. Mosby Co., 1990.)

*Total WBC/mm^3 by age in the normal child can be further delineated as follows (mean ± 2 SD): <6 wk: 3.7 ± 6.8; 6 wk–3 mo: 2.9 ± 5.7; 3 mo–6 mo: 1.9 ± 4.0; 6–12 mo: 2.6 ± 4.9; >12 mo: 1.9 ± 5.4.

†If Gram's stain is negative, a methylene blue stain may distinguish intracellular bacteria from nuclear material.

‡85% of partially treated patients will have a positive Gram's stain and >95% have positive cultures. Counterimmunoelectrophoresis (CIE) may be helpful if the culture is negative.

33 Ataxia

Ataxia is associated with impaired motor coordination, due to cerebellar dysfunction, without diminished motor strength. Afferent connections from the muscles, tendons, joints, and labyrinth may be dysfunctional due to either intrinsic cerebellar dysfunction or damage to peripheral nerves or spinal cord. Cerebellar dysfunction commonly produces unilateral disturbance of skilled movement; distal involvement is greater than proximal. Swaying of the trunk when sitting, standing, or walking may also be a predominant presentation. Sensory ataxia due to injury of a peripheral nerve or posterior spinal cord column is associated with a patient being able to stand with the feet together when the eyes are open but not when the eyes are closed (positive Romberg's sign).

Etiologic Considerations

A host of infectious, traumatic, and toxicologic conditions produce ataxia. Congenital (Freidreich's ataxia, ataxia telangiectasia) and metabolic conditions (Hartnup's, maple syrup urine disease) have insidious onset of ataxia associated with progression.

Life-threatening causes of ataxia are meningitis, posterior fossa tumor, cerebellar or posterior fossa hemorrhage, and hydrocephalus.

Diagnostic Approach

1. *Historically*, a careful delineation of the nature of neurological and associated findings must be defined (Table 33-1).
   a. Progression, acuteness, recurrent nature of neurologic signs and symptoms with respect to dizziness, weakness, vertigo, headache.
   b. Preceding events including trauma, ingestion of drugs, infection, respiratory symptoms. Family history should be explored.
2. *Physical examination* includes a complete neurologic assessment. In the infant, observation, watching the child in natural activities, is crucial.
   a. Specific examination of cerebellar function as well as mental status, motor strength, and sensory deficit. Look for nystagmus, incoordination, swaying, walking difficulty, or obvious dizziness. The Romberg sign as well as finger-to-nose and heel-to-shin are useful.
   b. An otolaryngologic examination may be appropriate.
3. *Diagnostic work-up* should include a search for specific etiologic conditions.
   a. Toxin levels, if any history of ingestion or exposure.
   b. Lumbar puncture for infectious or inflammatory process.
   c. CT scan to exclude mass or increased intracranial pressure.

   Alert: Acute onset of ataxia requires an extensive evaluation of differential considerations.

Table 33-1. Ataxia: Etiologic Considerations

Condition	Diagnostic Findings	Comments
Infection/Inflammation		
Acute cerebellar ataxia	Prodrome fever, respiratory, GI illness; rapid onset; transient cerebellar ataxia; normal mental function; CSF: normal or lymphocytosis	2–6-year-olds; transient; usually viral
Encephalitis/meningitis (Chap. 32)	Fever, toxicity, altered mental status; may be post infectious; cerebellar ataxia; CSF: increased protein and WBCs, decreased glucose	Usually resolves following adequate treatment
Acute labyrinthitis/ sinusitis	Vertigo, cerebellar ataxia, nystagmus, tinnitus, hearing loss, headache	May accompany otitis, trauma
Multiple sclerosis	Cerebellar ataxia; spastic weakness, optic neuritis, diplopia, variable neurologic deficits; CSF: increased cells, protein	Relapsing
Intoxication		
Phenytoin	Cerebellar ataxia, nystagmus	Level > 30 μg/ml
Lead	Anorexia, vomiting, lethargy, cerebellar ataxia	Also mercury and thallium
Carbon monoxide	Headache, confusion, exposure	CO level > 30 mg%
Alcohol	Cerebellar ataxia; slurred speech, progressive impaired mentation	
Trauma		
Head trauma Cerebellar hemorrhage Posterior fossa Subdural hematoma	Head trauma, headache, variable mental status; cerebellar ataxia; CT scan abnormal	
Heat stroke/exhaustion	Fatigue, weakness, progressive mental status deterioration; febrile; cerebellar ataxia	Excessive heat exposure
Psychiatric		
Hysteria	Inconsistent findings	Stress, mental illness

Bibliography

Cotton DG: Acute cerebellar ataxia. Arch Dis Child 32:181, 1957.

Stumpf DA: The inherited ataxias. Neuro Clin 3:47, 1985.

34 Headache

Pain sensitive structures in the head are either extracranial (paranasal and mastoid sinuses, orbits, teeth, scalp, and neck muscles) or intracranial (dura mater, venous sinuses, vessels of the pia-arachnoid). The brain parenchyma, ependymal linings of the ventricles, and meninges are not generally pain sensitive.

(See also p. 261.)

Etiologic Considerations

Headaches result from a variety of etiologic conditions, reflecting a variety of mechanisms (Table 34-1).

1. Muscle contraction.
   a. Tension.
2. Vascular.
   a. Migraine.
   b. Cluster.
   c. Hypertension.
3. Inflammatory.
   a. Meningitis.
   b. Sinusitis.
   c. Dental abscess.
4. Traction.
   a. Increased intracranial pressure (cerebral edema, neoplasm, hydrocephalus, hemorrhage).
   b. Lumbar puncture.
5. Other.
   a. Post-traumatic.
   b. Psychogenic (depression, conversion).

Diagnostic Approach

1. *History* must focus on excluding organic and psychosocial entities while describing the nature of the headaches in detail.
   a. Characterize the headache.
      (1) Temporal pattern: acute (single event with no previous episodes), acute and recurrent, chronic and progressive (suggestive of potential increased intracranial pressure with increasing severity and frequency), or chronic and nonprogressive (several times per day or week with no change in severity or accompanying signs and symptoms).
      (2) Preceding aura, scotomata, tingling, numbness.
      (3) Location of pain.

Table 34-1. Headache: Etiologic Considerations

Condition	Diagnostic Findings	Comments
Meningitis/encephalitis (Chap. 32)	Acute onset, infectious prodrome; localization reflects meningeal irritation; pain on movement; diffuse headache; lumbar puncture diagnostic	Support, antibiotics, hospitalize
Sinusitis	Unilateral or bilateral localized headache; pain on percussion; purulent rhinorrhea; ethmoid sinusitis: pain behind eyes to temporal/occipital areas; frontal sinusitis: pain above inner canthus of eye	X-rays or CT scan; antibiotics; associated ENT conditions; drainage
Dental abscess	Localized abscess, tenderness	Dental referral
Vascular		
Migraine	Unilateral, recurrent headache; prodromal findings of photophobia, nausea, vomiting, facial flushing, abdominal pain, transient blindness; scotomata, hemianopsia, paresthesias uncommon in children; complicated-ophthalmoplegia, hemiplegic, basilar	Rare in children under 7; often stress related; GI problems rare; positive family history (25–50%)
Cluster	Paroxysmal, sudden, orbital or frontal headache; unilateral autonomic symptoms—lacrimation, nasal stuffiness, Horner's syndrome	Rare in children; lasts 30–120 min with recurrence in 24 hr
Hypertension (Chap. 12)	Diffuse headache, nausea, vomiting, confusion, focal neurologic finding; high BP; exclude intracranial bleed	Unusual; underlying illness: glomerulonephritis, cardiac, etc.
Trauma (Chap. 47)		
Concussion/postconcussive	Diffuse headache following trauma; often accompanying dizziness, confusion, sensitivity to noise, emotional instability; neurologically normal; CT scan	Observe with frequent exams; exclude subdural or epidural hematoma, fracture
Muscle contraction	Muscle tenderness, tightening, especially in neck area; worse in afternoon	Usually related to stress

Table 34-1. Headache: Etiologic Considerations (*continued*)

Intoxication		
Carbon monoxide	Headache, weakness, dizziness, coma; carboxyhemoglobin level	Exposure history, improves with oxygen, removal from source
Lead/heavy metal	Diffuse headache, weakness, irritability, personality change, ataxia, red cell-aminolevulinic acid dehydratase	Exposure history; pica
Neoplasm		
Cerebral/cerebellar	Headache, vomiting, ataxia, papilledema, increased intracranial pressure marked by awakening at night, associated with vomiting and worsening with position	Rapid evaluation including CT; intervention
Pseudotumor cerebri	Generalized headache, full fontanelle, nausea, vomiting, diplopia, variable papilledema, increased intracranial pressure	Predisposing factors: viral illness, intoxication, steroids, head trauma, etc.
Miscellaneous		
Eye-Refractive error	Generalized headache; improves with glasses	
Eye-Glaucoma	Generalized headache, blurred vision	
High altitude	Diffuse headache, weakness	Recent altitude change
Temporomandibular joint (TMJ) disease	Pain with mandibular movement, pressure; frontal/temporal pain	Often related to stress
S/P lumbar puncture	Diffuse headache following procedure	Rare in children

(4) Nature of the pain described as steady, intermittent, throbbing, dull, pressure, or sharp. Severity of the pain with respect to interference with activities, response to simple analgesia, rest, or position.

(5) Migraine headaches often have accompanying eye, motor, or gastrointestinal findings.

b. Preceding events including stress (environment, school, arguments, fear), noise, fatigue, and trauma.

c. Preceding illness such as viral syndrome, gastroenteritis, sinusitis, ear infection, or preexisting contributing conditions including pica, ingestions, exposures, medications, hypertension, heart disease, and seizures.

d. Family history of migraines, headaches, and stress.

e. History of depression, school phobia, and recent trauma.

2. *Physical examination* should focus on neurologic assessment and contributing conditions.

a. A careful neurological evaluation is essential, including visual acuity, cerebellar signs, and auscultation for bruits.

b. Assessment of respiratory tract, sinuses, ears, eyes, and other findings.

c. Search for muscle pain, spasm, or tenderness.

3. *Diagnostic work-up* may not be needed if the history and physical examination suggest a nonorganic cause. If a work-up is indicated, studies should include laboratory and radiology.

a. Laboratory

(1) Lumbar puncture (meningismus)

(2) Electroencephalogram (paroxysmal, recurrent headache)

b. Radiology

(1) CT scan (elevated intracranial pressure, progressive or new neurological findings, focal EEG, meningismus, or partial seizure).

(2) Radiographs of skull (trauma) and sinuses (point tenderness, pressure sensitive).

Alert: Rapid onset of severe disabling headache usually requires expeditious evaluation.

Bibliography

Cooper PJ, Bawden HN, Camfield PR, et al.: Anxiety and life events in childhood migraine. Pediatrics 79:999, 1987.

Prensky AL: Migraine and migrainous variants in pediatric patients. Pediatr Clin North Am 23:461, 1976.

Shinnar S and D'Souza BJ: Diagnosis and management of headache in children. Pediatr Clin North Am 29:79, 1981.

35 Paralysis

Paralysis may often present as a partial deficit associated with difficulty with walking as well as with more complete motor abnormalities. Flaccid paralysis is accompanied by motor weakness and absent or diminished deep reflexes (Table 35-1).

Etiologic Considerations

See Table 35-1.

Diagnostic Approach

1. *Historical* data should focus on defining the nature of the loss and potential contributing conditions.
   a. Nature of motor weakness or loss: progression, remission, recurrence, involvement.
   b. Recent infectious illness, fever, viral prodrome, and immunization, tick exposure, trauma, ingestion, vascular disorder.
2. *Physical examination* must include a complete neurological exam.
   a. Degree of motor loss, distribution, associated cranial nerves and sensory changes.
   b. Associated findings.
   c. Defining sensory losses using dermatomes may be helpful.
3. *Diagnostic work-up* should be individualized.
   a. Blood studies as indicated.
   b. Lumbar puncture.
   c. CT scan, plain films of spine.

   Alert: Organic etiology may be defined, using the pattern of paralysis and consistency with specific neurologic distribution. Associated signs and symptoms may assist in defining the cause.

Bibliography

Burse GS and Strauss RW: Acute childhood hemiplegia. Ann Emerg Medc 14:74, 1985.

Gold AP and Carter S: Acute hemiplegia of infancy and childhood. Pediatr Clin North Am 23:413, 1976.

Table 35-1. Paralysis: Etiologic Considerations

Conditions	Diagnostic Findings	Comments
Infection/Inflammatory		
Viral encephalitis (Chap. 32)	Altered mental status; transient, progressive	Herpes, coxsackievirus
Poliomyelitis	Prodrome fever, respiratory, GI findings; flaccid asymmetric paralysis, lower extremities, bulbar involvement; muscle pain, tenderness, fasciculations; CSF: pleocytosis	Prevent with vaccine
Guillain-Barré syndrome	Nonspecific respiratory, GI findings; symmetric flaccid paralysis, greater proximally; CSF: elevated protein	Unknown etiology
Tick-bite paralysis	Muscle pain and paresthesia, ascending flaccid symmetric paralysis 1 week after bite	Toxin release by tick
Secondary polyneuropathy	Low grade fever, systemic illness; variable flaccid paralysis with loss of DTR, position, vibration; ataxia	Viral and bacterial (botulism, diphtheria) infections, autoimmune, immunization, poisoning
Transverse myelitis	Rapid progression, ataxia, weakness, multiple neurologic deficits; optic neuritis; paralysis with sensory loss below lesion, hyperesthesia above	Unknown etiology; may be related to multiple sclerosis
Trauma		
Blunt trauma to neck	Variable findings depending upon level of injury	Fracture, dislocation
Penetrating trauma	Immediate or delayed findings	
Vascular		
Congenital heart disease Endocarditis Dysrhythmias Arteriovenous malformation	Variable findings reflecting nature of emboli, mass effect; systemic disease; CT scan and evaluation of underlying disease	Embolic phenomenon
Sickle cell disease	Variable findings	Thrombosis, spasm
Hemophilia	Large joints, CNS, spinal bleed	Acute mass effect
Hemiplegic migraine	Headache with prodrome and accompanying paralysis	

Table 35-1. Paralysis: Etiologic Considerations (*continued*)

Conditions	Diagnostic Findings	Comments
Other		
Todd's paralysis (Chap. 36)	Transient paralysis following seizure; resolves	
Metabolic	Variable	Hypo-/hyperkalemia; rhabdomyolysis, porphyria

36 Seizures (Convulsions)

A seizure is a paroxysmal abnormality of nerve cells producing motor, sensory, autonomic, or psychic disturbance (Table 36-1).

(See also p. 249.)

Etiologic Considerations

Age and pattern of onset have a significant impact on diagnostic considerations.

1. First day of life.
   a. Hypoxia.
   b. Drugs or intoxication.
   c. Trauma.
   d. Infection.
   e. Metabolic: hyper-/hypoglycemia, pyridoxine deficiency.
2. Second and third days of life.
   a. Infection.
   b. CNS malformation.
   c. Metabolic: hyper-/hyponatremia, hypocalcemia, hypoglycemia, inborn errors.
3. One to six months of life.
   a. Infection.
   b. CNS malformation.
   c. Metabolic: hypocalcemia, hyponatremia, inborn errors.
4. Six months to three years.
   a. Febrile seizure.
   b. Infection.
   c. Trauma.
   d. CNS disorder.
   e. Intoxication.
   f. Metabolic.
5. Older children.
   a. Idiopathic epilepsy (often with poor compliance).
   b. Infection.
   c. Trauma.
   d. CNS disorder.

Febrile seizures are by far the most common cause of seizures in children between 5 months and 5 years of age. Infection, trauma, poor compliance (in patients on anticonvulsants for epilepsy), intoxication, and idiopathic epilepsy are the other most common acute cause. Epilepsy accounts for most chronic disease.

A number of conditions may simulate seizures and must be clinically distinguished. In the *infant*, consider apnea, tremor, micturitional shivering, and dysrhythmias while the *child*, breath-holding, micturitional/coughing syncope, migraines, and night tremors should be excluded. *Adolescents* may hyperventilate or become hysterical, experience vasomotor syncope, pseudoseizures, orthostatic hypotension, or micturitional/cough syncope.

Table 36-1. Seizures: Etiologic Considerations

Condition	Diagnostic Findings	Comments
Infection		
Febrile seizure	Fever, grand mal seizure; CSF: normal	5 mo–5 yr; self-limited; most common cause; fever reflects underlying illness
Meningitis/encephalitis (Chap. 32)	Fever, headache, toxicity, Kernig's, Brudzinsky's, bulging fontanelle; CSF: diagnostic	Viral or bacterial; may be epidemic
S/P immunization	History of immunization	DTP, measles, etc.
Pertussis, rabies, tetanus, syphilis	Disease specific findings	
Trauma (Chap. 47)		
Concussion	Trauma followed by variable abnormal exam; focal or grand mal seizure; CT scan normal	May be recurrent
Subdural hematoma	Change in mentation with progression; CT scan abnormal	
Epidural hematoma	Lucid period following trauma followed by impaired mentation; CT	
Birth hypoxia	History of perinatal injury; low Apgar, premature	
Psychiatric		
Breath-holding	Breath-holding precipitated by crying, anger, injury followed by loss of consciousness; seizures rare and self-limited	6 mo–4 yr; cyanosis precedes loss of consciousness; in seizures, consciousness lost first; may mimic seizure
Hyperventilation	Tachypnea	
Hysteria	Anxious, stressed	May mimic seizure
Endocrine/Metabolic		
Hypoglycemia (Chap. 31)	Pallor, sweating, syncope	< 40 mg/dl in child, < 30 mg/dl in term infant
Hypo-/hypernatremia	Listless, irritable, associated condition	Dehydration, inappropriate ADH
Hypocalcemia	Muscle cramps, pain, Chvostek's, Trousseau's	Parathyroid deficiency, premature
Hypomagnesemia	Tetany, tremor, irritability	
Inborn errors of metabolism	Neurologically abnormal, delayed development	Phenylketonuria, amino/organic acidemia
Uremia	Evidence of renal failure	

Table 36-1. Seizures: Etiologic Considerations (*continued*)

Condition	Diagnostic Findings	Comments
Intoxication		
Aspirin, amphetamine, anticholinergics, theophylline, CO, PCP, cocaine, alcohol	Signs and symptoms associated with drug intoxication or withdrawal	
Other		
Birth asphyxia	Perinatal injury, low Apgar	Infection, placental insufficiency
Neurocutaneous syndrome	Skin findings, variable neuro exam, family history; CT scan	
Degenerative/deficiency	Variable	Pyridoxine deficiency, Tay Sachs, etc.
Neoplasm	Variable	Glioma, most common
Hypertensive encephalopathy (Chap. 12)	High blood pressure, vomiting, ataxia, facial paralysis	May be secondary to stroke or renal

Diagnostic Approach

1. *History* must focus on the nature of the seizure (Table 36-2) and related findings.
   a. Past history of neurologic disease, seizures, breath holding, metabolic, or endocrine disease.
   b. Type of seizure, length, response to therapy. Focal or generalized.
   c. Response to therapy.
   d. Associated fever or febrile illness, trauma, intoxication, renal disease, vomiting, diarrhea, anxiety, or stress.
2. *Physical examination.*
   a. Complete neurologic examination after stabilization.
   b. Examination to search for underlying illness.
3. *Diagnostic work-up.*
   a. Chemistry should include a glucose (bedside technique adequate). Electrolytes, Ca^{++}, Mg^{++}, and PO_4^- indicated if there is a history of abnormal intake or output, endocrinologic, or renal disease. Other studies as indicated by specific conditions.
   b. CBC and urinalysis in the febrile patient.
   c. Lumbar puncture should be performed in febrile patients who are young (under 12–18 months of age), have abnormal neurologic examinations or complex, unusual seizure patterns. Analysis of the spinal fluid should include culture and Gram's stain, protein and glucose, and cell count (see Table 32-2).
   d. Drug levels to measure anticonvulsant levels (if currently taking) or to exclude intoxication.
   e. An electroencephalogram (EEG) is indicated to assess electrical activity. The study may be useful in defining the site, type, and nature of a seizure disorder. Nonspecific background changes may persist for 1–6 weeks after any type of seizure and are not diagnostic.
   f. Radiologic studies to exclude intracranial disease, especially intracranial mass. CT scan is diagnostic.

Alert: Seizures result from a range of conditions necessitating a thorough history and physical supplemented by laboratory data. Management of airway is essential if the seizure is prolonged, followed by consideration of administration of glucose and narcan. Diagnostic studies are necessary.

Table 36-2. Common Types of Seizures

Type	Etiology	Diagnostic Findings
Grand Mal (tonic clonic)	Idiopathic, genetic, infection, intoxication, trauma, metabolic	Aura: motor, sensory (smell), visceral (abdominal pain), tonic (stiffening)-clonic (rhythmic jerking); incontinence
Psychomotor, complex partial	Idiopathic, hypoxia, trauma, infection	Aura: fever, abdominal pain; automatism: rubbing, chewing, staring; psychic, numbness, tingling
Petit mal (absence)	Idiopathic, genetic	No aura, transient (5–20 sec) lapse, staring, not postictal

Bibliography

Delgado-Escueta AV, Aicardi J, Rey E, et al.: Management of status epilepticus. N Engl J Med 306:1337, 1982.

Nelson KB and Ellenberg JH: Prognosis in children with febrile seizures. Pediatrics 61:720, 1978.

Simon R: Physiologic consequences of status epilepticus. Epilepsia 26 (S 1):558, 1985.

37 Syncope (Fainting)

Syncope, or fainting, is the transient, sudden loss of consciousness accompanied by loss of postural tone and falling due to cerebral hypoxia. No prodromal symptoms are noted and there is a rapid return to the premorbid mental status. Although in children and adolescents the cause is usually a benign condition, vascular, infectious, and cardiac conditions must be considered.

Etiologic Considerations

Fainting is most commonly associated with anxiety or hysteria due to a vasomotor event. It is essential to distinguish syncope from *dizziness*, which is not associated with any change in consciousness or incontinence. *Seizures* are differentiated by prolonged (> 5 min) alteration in mentation, accompanying tonic-clonic movements, and incontinence followed by a period of confusion or listlessness (Table 37-1).

Diagnostic Approach

1. *Historical* data should determine the nature of the incident.
   a. A careful description of the event, including rapidity of onset and progression, the duration, loss of consciousness, incontinence, and associated signs and symptoms.
   b. Prodromal signs and symptoms, precipitating and predisposing factors, recent psychiatric disturbances, intoxication, and post-syncopal findings.
   c. Past medical problems, metabolic abnormalities, social interactions, and family history.
2. *Physical examination* allows for exclusion of certain entities.
   a. Vital signs, including orthostatics.
   b. Cardiovascular and pulmonary examination focusing on aortic disease, dysrhythmias, and so on.
   c. Neurologic examination.
3. *Diagnostic work-up* should be specific for the history and physical; these additional studies are not always required.
   Laboratory.
   a. CBC, electrolytes, glucose, toxicologic screens.
   b. ECG, rhythm strip, and monitoring if any concern about dysrhythmia.
   c. EEG to exclude seizure disorder.

Alert: Syncope in children is rarely associated with significant cardiac or pulmonary disease but life-threatening abnormalities must be excluded.

Table 37-1. Syncope: Etiologic Considerations

Condition	Diagnostic Findings	Comment
Psychiatric		
Vasovagal	Rapid drop in blood pressure; accompanying nausea, vomiting, sweating, pallor, blurred vision, weakness; self-limited	Precipitated by fear, pain, anxiety, noxious stimuli; usually in hot, humid, closed space; common in adolescents
Hyperventilation	Rapid, deep respirations; weakness, tingling, numbness of hands	Response to anxiety, stress; responds to rebreathing
Breath holding	Cyanosis and unconsciousness following vigorous crying; usually self-limited	Triggered by crying, anger, upset; usually in infancy; rare hypoxic seizure
Hysteria	Anxiety; avoids injury	Responds to environmental stimulus, decreased mentation
Vascular		
Postural hypotension	Episode following prolonged recumbent position with subsequent rising	Secondary poor cerebral perfusion; avoid rapid position change
Heart problems Congenital or acquired	Cardiac murmur, low output with poor perfusion, pallor	Secondary poor cerebral perfusion
Congestive heart failure (CHF) or dysrhythmias (Chap. 11)	Tachypnea, dyspnea, tachycardia, cardiomegaly, diaphoresis, cyanosis	Secondary poor cerebral perfusion
Infection		
Upper airway obstruction (Chap. 46)		
Croup Epiglottitis	Stridor, labored respirations; variably toxic, febrile	Secondary poor cerebral perfusion
Lower airway disease (Chap. 46)		
Pneumonia	Tachypnea, ronchi, fever, respiratory distress	Secondary poor cerebral perfusion
Allergy		
Asthma Anaphylaxis	Tachypnea, wheezing, cough	Secondary poor cerebral perfusion
Intoxication		
Alcohol Anticholinergic Antidepressants Cholinergic Hallucinogens Narcotics/sedatives Sympathomimetics	History of overdose; hypotension, dysrhythmia, poor peripheral perfusion; variable associated findings	Variable mechanisms

Table 37-1. *(continued)*

Condition	Diagnostic Findings	Comment
Metabolic		
Hypoglycemia (Chap. 31) Hypo-/hypernatremia	Pallor, sweating, nausea, vomiting, tachycardia, tachypnea, dysrhythmia	Secondary cerebral hypoglycemia, poor perfusion
Trauma		
Foreign body	Stridor, respiratory distress, other findings	Secondary poor cerebral perfusion
Miscellaneous		
Epilepsy (Chap. 36)	Tonic-clonic seizure or transient loss of consciousness; incontience, postictal period	History, EEG helpful
Dehydration (Chap. 4)	Hypotension (orthostatic), poor peripheral perfusion	Secondary poor cerebral perfusion
Posttussive/ postmicturition	Episode following event	Secondary poor cerebral perfusion
Anemia (Chap. 29)	Pale, tachycardia, dizzy	Decreased oxygen carrying capacity
High altitude barotrauma	Rapid change altitude, tachypnea	Relative cerebral hypoxia

Bibliography

Gordon RA, Moodie DS, Passalacqua M, et al.: A retrospective analysis of the cost-effective work-up of syncope in children. Cleve Clin Q 54:931, 1987.

Missri J, Alexander S: Hyperventilation syndrome. JAMA 240:2093, 1978.

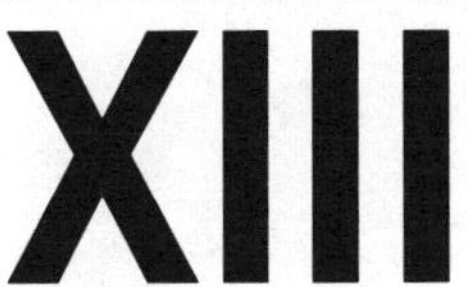

XIII Orthopedic Problems

38 Arthralgia and Joint Pain

Pain, swelling, and joint discomfort accompany arthralgia. If the joint is inflamed with accompanying redness, warmth, swelling, and pain, the patient has arthritis.

Etiologic Considerations

Not all arthralgia has accompanying arthritis. It is essential to define the joints involved in considering diagnostic entities (Table 38-1).

Also see Chap. 39.

Diagnostic Approach

1. *History* is essential in differentiating various entities. Hip pain may be referred to the knee.
   a. Nature of the joint discomfort or pain.
      (1) Duration and progression of pain.
      (2) Activities that worsen or improve the pain.
      (3) Joints involved.
      (4) Previous episodes of arthralgia with pattern of reoccurrence.
   b. Associated signs and symptoms, especially GI, renal, neurologic findings.
   c. Preexisting medical conditions, trauma, or family history.
2. *Physical examination* must define the type of joint involvement present.
   a. Joint examination of all joints for swelling, warmth, fluid, tenderness, and range of motion.
   b. Careful assessment for other systemic findings.
   c. Neurologic and motor evaluation.
3. *Diagnostic work-up*.
   a. Laboratory.
      (1) CBC, ESR if any suggestion of infectious or inflammatory disease. If a fever or elevated ESR (> 30 mm/hr) is present, an infectious or inflammatory process is 8 times more likely than if both are absent. If both are present, only 7% of these patients lack an inflammatory or infectious process.
      (2) Joint aspirate to determine cell count, glucose, and protein.
      (3) ANA and rheumatoid factor are variably positive.
      (4) Bacteriologic studies may be useful if bacterial infection is suggested (e.g., septic arthritis, osteomyelitis). Joint or bone aspirates are valuable. Evaluation of fluid beyond culture and Gram's stain should also include cell count, glucose, and mucin clot or string test.
   b. Radiologic plain film x-rays and bone scans may be useful. Follow-up plain films are often useful, given that callus or periosteal reaction may not be present for 7–10 days in patients with hairline fractures or osteomyelitis.
   c. Therapeutic trial of inflammatory induced disease may often benefit from aspirin, especially if juvenile rheumatoid arthritis is a consideration.

Table 38-1. Arthralgia: Etiologic Considerations

Condition	Joint	Diagnostic Findings
Trauma		
Sprain Fracture	Usually monoarticular	History of trauma; joint tenderness, swelling; impaired movement; fracture may be occult, requiring follow-up x-ray; exclude nonaccidental trauma
Infection		
Toxic synovitis of hip	Hip	Preceding viral illness without systemic toxicity; often presents with limp; hip rarely warm, tender; limited range of motion; CBC, ESR normal; x-ray: variable effusion
Septic, arthritis	Monoarticular	Acute onset fever, toxicity with local tenderness, warmness, swelling: CBC, ESR elevated; x-ray: effusion; may need bone scan or joint aspiration; requires emergent intervention
Arthritis, miscellaneous	Variable	Local swelling, warmth, tenderness; associated findings (rubella, hepatitis, Ebstein-Barr virus, chickenpox, tuberculosis, fungi, syphilis)
Osteomyelitis	Monoarticular, long bones (tibia, femur)	Fever, variable toxicity; local swelling, tenderness, warmth; CBC, ESR elevated; x-ray: swelling, periosteal elevation, lytic lesion; bone scan positive; bone aspiration
Inflammatory		
Juvenile rheumatoid		
Acute febrile (20% JRA)	Variable; 25% severe	Irritable, listless, hyperpyrexia, maculopapular rash; elevated CBC, ESR; ANA, rheumatoid factor negative; trial aspirin
Polyarticular (30% JRA)	≥ 4 joints (knee, ankle, wrist, elbow, hand)	Anorexia, listless, low-grade fever, rare rash, iridocyclitis; elevated CBC, ESR; ANA (25%), rheumatoid factor (15%) positive; trial aspirin or steroids
Monoarticular (50% JRA)	Monoarticular (knee common)	Swollen, tender in morning; CBC, ESR normal; ANA (25%), rheumatoid factor rarely positive
Rheumatic fever	Migratory, polyarticular (knee, ankle, wrist, elbow)	Swollen, red, tender, painful; carditis, chorea, nodule, erythema marginatum, fever; variable CBC; elevated ESR, streptozyme; trial aspirin

Henoch-Schonlein purpura	Migratory, polyarthritis (large joints)	Swollen, tender; purpuric rash lower extremity (ankles, buttock) extending upward; abdominal pain, diarrhea, nephritis
Inflammatory bowel disease	Polyarthritis (large joints)	Swollen, tender; diarrhea, abdominal pain, rectal bleeding; sigmoidoscopy, barium enema
Congenital		
Hemophilia	Monoarticular	Swollen, tender; history hemophilia, abnormal bleeding
Sickle cell	Polyarticular	Systemic disease; positive Sickledex
Dislocated hip	Monoarticular	Unstable joint; positive Ortolani's sign; x-ray abnormal
Miscellaneous		
Legg-Calvé-Perthes	Hip	Limited range movement; may be referred to knee; x-ray: bulging capsule, wide space; peak in males 4–10 yr; avascular necrosis proximal femoral head
Slipped capital femoral epiphysis	Unilateral or bilateral hips	Limited abduction, internal rotation; worse with activity; usually obese or tall child; x-ray: widening epiphyseal growth plate
Osteochondritis dissecans	Knee	Painful, stiff with effusion; x-ray: demineralization medial femoral condyle
Neoplasm	Variable	

Alert: If there is any question of a septic arthritis, it must be evaluated expeditiously.

Bibliography

Kunnamo I, Kallio P, Pelkonen P, et al.: Clinical signs and laboratory tests in the differential diagnosis of arthritis in children. Am J Dis Child 141:34, 1987.

Kunnamo I and Pelkonen P: Routine analysis of synovial fluid cells is of value in the differential diagnosis of arthritis in children. J Rheumatol 13:1076, 1986.

39 Limp

Gait disturbances produce a limp associated with an abnormality of rhythm, usually caused by pain. About 15% of school-aged children without a history of chronic disease may have limb pain at some time. About 4% of these children report having had extra-articular limb pain or pain significant enough to alter routine activity.

Etiologic Considerations

Limp may result from painful or painless conditions. Referred pain may occur, a painful knee often being related to actual hip disease while hip complaints can occur with abdominal or spinal pathology (Table 39-1).

By age group, conditions most commonly noted with limping include:

1. *1–5 years.*
   a. Toxic synovitis.
   b. Occult fracture.
   c. Osteomyelitis.
   d. Septic arthritis.
   e. Juvenile rheumatoid arthritis.
2. *5–10 years.*
   a. Toxic synovitis.
   b. Legg-Calvé-Perthes disease.
3. *10–15 years.*
   a. Slipped capital femoral epiphysis.
   b. Osgood-Schlatter disease.
   c. Osteochondroses.

Also see Chap. 38.

Diagnostic Approach

1. *History* should focus on the progression, nature of the limp, associated signs and symptoms, and preexisting problems.
   a. Onset and progression of the gait abnormality. Pain, weakness, limited range of movement, type (large or small) of joints involved, tenderness, swelling, and point discomfort.
   b. History of trauma, fever, other joint and bone involvement, and preexisting problems.
   c. Signs and symptoms related to the involved extremity.
   d. Associated systemic signs and symptoms including motor and sensory deficits, incontinence, loss of weight, and fever.
2. *Physical examination* should focus on the involved area.
   a. Careful examination of involved areas and those distant for tenderness, warmth, erythema, swelling, fluid, and range of motion.
   b. Careful neurological examination.
   c. Other involved areas and systemic findings.

Table 39-1. Limp: Etiologic Considerations

Conditions	Diagnostic Findings	Ancillary Data	Comments
Infection/Inflammatory			
Toxic synovitis of hip	Acute or insidious onset; hip rarely warm, tender, or with limited range motion	CBC, ESR; hip x-ray: variable effusion	Studies often normal; aspirate if any question of infection
Osteomyelitis	Local swelling, tenderness, warmth, monoarticular, long bones; variable fever toxicity	CBC, ESR; x-ray, technetium bone scan; joint or bone aspirate	Important to exclude
Septic arthritis	Acute onset, tender, warm, limited range of motion; monoarticular; variable fever	CBC, ESR; x-ray, scan; joint aspirate	Aspirate is diagnostic; GC may be migratory
Arthritis Viral Mycobacterium Hepatitis Vaccine (rubella)	Subacute or insidious; polyarticular, variable associated symptoms	CBC, ESR; x-ray; joint aspirate	Variable course, reflecting etiology
Appendicitis			
Diskitis	Tenderness, nonspecific discomfort with walking	CBC, ESR; x-ray, CT of spine	Etiology, treatment uncertain
Polio	Asymmetric flaccid paralysis, bulbar involved	CSF pleocytosis; viral culture	Unusual
Guillain-Barré	Ascending symmetric paralysis with pain and paresthesias; cranial nerve involvement	CSF: high protein	Respiratory insufficiency

Trauma			
Sprain/contusion	History trauma, local pain, tenderness, swelling, ecchymosis	X-ray normal	Support, follow
Fracture	Variable trauma, pain, tenderness, swelling; may be occult	X-ray positive; if negative, do serial studies	Immobilize, follow
Foreign body/splinter	Acute onset pain, local swelling, erythema	X-ray if radioopaque	Remove
Poorly fitting shoe	Limp disappears when shoe removed		
Vertebral disk injury	Motor, sensory, reflex defect	X-ray	Consultation
Vascular			
Legg-Calvé-Perthes	Insidious onset pain of hip with limp/limitation in motion	X-ray: bulging capsule with widened joint space	Peak: Male (4:1) 4–10 yr; treat abduction/internal rotation
Degenerative			
Slipped capital femoral epiphysis	Unilateral/bilateral pain knee (referred) or medial aspect thigh; limitation of abduction and internal rotation	X-ray: widened epiphyseal growth plate	Obese/tall-thin child, 12–15 yr; surgical immobilization
Osgood-Schlatter	Pain knee caused by patellar tendonitis as insertion into tibial tubercle	X-ray: fragmentation tibial tuberosity	Peak: 11–15 yr; support
Osteochondroses	Irregularity of involved bone	X-ray: WNL	Teenagers; support
Congenital			
Hemophilia	Variable history trauma; muscle bleed, monoarticular joint swelling	X-ray; variable bleeding screen	Factor replacement
Sickle Cell	Bone pain, polyarticular joint involvement	X-ray; Hct, positive sickle cell prep	May be crisis or infarct

Table 39-1. Limp: Etiologic Considerations (*continued*)

Conditions	Diagnostic Findings	Ancillary Data	Comments
Dislocated hip	Unstable and limited range of hip motion; hip click	X-ray	Splint in flexion/abduction
Testicular torsion Incarcerated hernia	Acute onset of scrotal or groin pain; mass is tender, swollen		Surgical emergency
Autoimmune (Chap. 38)			
Neoplasm			
Ostochondroma	Local pain with exostosis		
Leukemia Neuroblastoma Ewing Spinal cord	Systemic disease with associated findings		
Miscellaneous			
Attention getting	Inconsistent signs and symptoms		May follow physical problem

3. *Diagnostic work-up.*

a. Laboratory evaluation should exclude systemic disease. If appropriate,

(1) Complete blood cell count (CBC) and sedimentation rate (ESR).

(2) Cultures and aspirates.

b. Radiologic evaluation of involved area and all potentially involved bones. If the initial study is normal, serial films over two weeks may demonstrate callus formation or other abnormalities. Look especially for buckle fractures in the cortex of the tibia, fibula, or femur. Rarely, technetium bone scans may be required to exclude early osteomyelitis or fracture.

Alert: Septic arthritis, osteomyelitis, and fracture must be excluded to assure that no medical emergency exists.

Bibliography

Barton LL, Dunkle LM, and Habib FH: Septic arthritis in children. Am J Dis Child 145:898, 1987.

Eichenwald HF: Antimicrobial therapy in infants and children: update 1976–1985. J Pediatr 107:161, 337, 1985.

Illingworth CM: 128 limping children with no fracture, sprain, or obvious cause. Clin Pediatr 17:139, 1978.

McCarthy PL, Wasserman D, Spiesel SZ, et al.: Evaluation of arthritis and arthralgia in the pediatric patient. Clin Pediatr 19:183, 1980.

XIV Renal and Genitourinary Problems

40 Dysuria and Frequency

Dysuria, or painful urination, is caused by irritation of the mucosa of the bladder or urethra leading to contraction and pain. Increased *frequency* of voiding of small volumes of urine stems from incomplete emptying of the bladder due to inflammation or atony caused by sacral nerve cord damage (Table 40-1).

(See also p. 262.)

Etiologic Considerations

Infection is the most common cause of dysuria or frequency associated with cystitis or pyelonephritis (Table 40-2).

Also see Chap. 41.

Diagnostic Approach

1. *History* should focus on the nature of the complaint.
   a. Nature of the dysuria with respect to the onset, progression, and factors that alleviate it. Infants may be irritable while older children may cry, strain, or be resistant to voiding.
   b. Define frequency of voiding and associated findings. Other systemic diseases, such as diabetes, renal disease, or excessive fluid intake.
   c. Associated costovertebral (CVA) pain or tenderness, fever, toxicity, and abdominal pain. Patients with renal stones have excruciating unilateral pain.
   d. Recent blunt or penetrating trauma or chemical exposure.
   e. Past episodes of urinary tract infection.
2. *Physical examination* primarily focuses on the abdomen.
   a. Abdomen and genitalia should be examined carefully, looking for tenderness, CVA discomfort, and other specific findings. Exclude foreign body.
   b. Other findings associated with causative conditions.
   c. Neurological assessment.
   d. Cystoscopy if any question of neoplasm.
3. *Diagnostic work-up*.
   a. Laboratory evaluation of renal function.
      (1) Urinalysis, including particular attention to crystals, WBCs, RBCs, and casts.
      (2) Urine culture.
         (a) A clean catch midstream specimen (CCMS) is obtained after carefully cleaning the perineum.
         (b) Catheterization using feeding tube in infants and gradually using urinary catheter.

Table 40-1. Causes of Dysuria and Frequency

	Dysuria	Frequency
Infection		
Urinary tract infection (cystitis/pyelonephritis)	+	+
Urethritis	+	
Prostatitis	+	
Vulvovaginitis	+	
Renal stone	+	
Trauma		
Foreign body	+	
Blunt trauma (Chap. 40)	+	
Chemical irritation	+	+
Miscellaneous		
Water overload		+
Osmotic diuresis (diabetes mellitus, diuretic)		+
Renal tubular dysfunction (renal failure, diabetes insipidus)		+
Anxiety		+
Neoplasm	+	

Table 40-2. Dysuria and Frequency: Etiologic Considerations

Condition	Diagnostic Findings	Comments
Infection		
Urinary tract infection Cystitis Pyelonephritis	Dysuria, frequency, burning; if pyelo: toxic, CVA tenderness, abdominal discomfort; urine: pyuria, bacteruria, variable hematuria	Most frequent cause; radiographic evaluation if multiple infection or < 1 yr
Urethritis	Dysuria, urethral discharge; culture, Gram's stain	
Vulvovaginitis	Vaginal discharge, pruritus, variable abdominal tenderness, dysuria; culture	
Trauma		
Foreign body	Dysuria, history foreign body, hematuria; culture negative	Masturbation, local trauma
Chemical irritation	Dysuria; pyuria, hematuria; culture negative	Detergent, bubble bath, perfumed soaps
Miscellaneous		
Psychogenic Water overload	Frequency, water overload	Trial: withhold water
Diabetes mellitus	Frequency; no other urinary complaints; systemic disease; glucose, ketones, pH	Insulin, fluids, close monitoring

(c) Suprapubic aspiration.

Collection Method	Colony Forming units/ml		
	Uninfected	**Uninterpretable**	**Infected**
Suprapubic	< 10		≥ 10
Straight catheter	< 10^3		≥ 10^3
CCMS	10^3	10^3–10^5	≥ 10^5
Bag	< 10^3	10^3–10^5	≥ 10^5

(3) Urethal or vaginal discharge examination for WBCs and bacteria.
(4) BUN and creatinine. Other studies to exclude other conditions.
(5) Concentrating studies and intake/output evaluation if indicated by question of diabetes insipidus, water intoxication, and so on.

b. Radiologic evaluation of renal anatomy.
(1) Assessment is indicated if multiple urinary tract infections, first infection in male, or child < 1 yr. Obtain voiding cystourethrogram (VCUG) and if normal, do ultrasound. If VCUG abnormal, do intravenous pyelogram (IVP).
(2) IVP if renal stone to be excluded.

c. Therapeutic trial of Pyridium may be useful as urinary analgesic if cystitis or lower tract disease is primary condition pending culture and sensitivity.

Alert: Infectious origin should generally be excluded by adequate urinalysis and culture.

Bibliography

Durbin WA and Peter G: Management of urinary tract infections in infants and children. Pediatr Inf Dis 3:564, 1984.

Barkin SZ, Barkin RM, and Horgan JG: Radiologic evaluation after urinary tract infection. In Barkin RM (ed.): *The Emergently Ill Child*. Rockville: Aspen Pub Co., 1987.

Choi H, Snyder HM, and Duckett JW: Urolithiasis in childhood: current management. J Pediatr Surg 22:158, 1987.

Demetrion E, Emans SJ, and Masland RP: Dysuria in adolescent girls: urinary tract infection or vaginitis. Pediatrics 70:299, 1982.

Ogra P and Faden H: Urinary tract infection in childhood: an update. J Pediatr 106:1023, 1985.

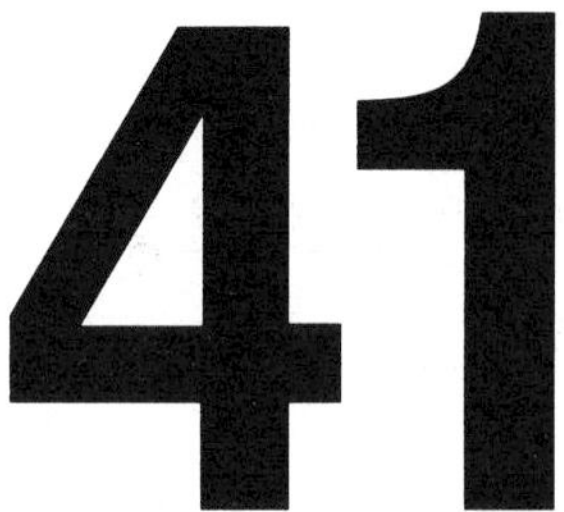

Hematuria and Proteinuria

Hematuria is present when there are ≥ 5 RBC/HPF in a sediment of 10 ml of centrifuged urine. Such microhematuria is often asymptomatic, resulting from nonrenal as well as glomerular and extraglomerular conditions. Gross hematuria is symptomatic.

Proteinuria is unequivocably present when over 200 mg/m^2/24 hr of protein is found in the urine. It is usually transient, occurring with fever, exercise, infection, CHF, or environmental stress. Orthostatic proteinuria occurs in an upright position, resolution being noted in 50% of individuals by early adulthood.

(See also Chap. 40.)

Etiologic Considerations

In focusing on diagnostic entities, it is essential to first determine if there is isolated hematuria or proteinuria, or concurrent presence of both (Table 41-1).

Hematuria in newborns is commonly due to vascular disorders such as hypoxia, thrombosis, or circulatory compromise. Urinary tract infections followed by glomerulonephritis and trauma are the important etiologies in older children.

Gross hematuria is common with infection, obvious perineal or meatal irritation, and trauma; tumor is a very rare cause. Etiologic distinctions in evaluating microscopic hematuria are based upon the presence of red blood cells, either free or as casts, or hemoglobin.

1. Free RBCs are commonly extraglomerular in origin reflecting:
   a. Infection.
   b. Trauma.
   c. GU malformation.
   d. Bleeding diathesis.
   e. Cystic disease.
   f. Instrumentation/iatrogenic.
   g. Drugs.
   h. Tumor.
   i. Calculi.
   j. Sickle cell disease.
2. RBC casts are indicative of a glomerular origin.
3. Hemoglobinuria or myoglobinuria is indicated with pigment casts and free or no RBC casts or free RBCs.
   a. Hemoglobinuria results from hemolytic anemias, incompatible blood transfusions, disseminated intravascular coagulation, infection (sepsis, malaria), hemolytic-uremic syndrome, drugs (carbon monoxide, sulfonamides), and snake venom.
   b. Myoglobinuria occurs with crush injuries, burns, myositis, and rhabdomyolysis.

The characteristics on page 189 help distinguish nonrenal from glomerular and extraglomerular pathology.

Table 41-1. Hematuria and Proteinuria: Etiologic Considerations

Condition	Diagnostic Finding	Hematuria	Proteinuria	Comments
Infection (nonrenal/ extraglomerular)				
Urinary tract infection	Fever, dysuria, frequency, burning; variable toxicity, CVA tenderess	Gross/micro	Positive	Cystitis, pyelonephritis; bacterial, viral, TB; culture, UA
Autoimmune (glomerular)				
Glomerulonephritis acute	Malaise, headache, oliguria, edema, hypertension	Gross/micro	Positive	Post-strep; low complement
Membranoproliferative	Insidious, headache, edema, hypertension	Gross/micro	Positive	Low complement; biopsy
Henoch-Schonlein	Purpuric rash, arthritis, GI involvement	Micro	Variable	Variable involvement
Nephrotic syndrome	Periorbital swelling, oliguria, edema, abdominal pain	Rare (25%)	Positive	Low albumin, high lipid; variable etiologies
Trauma (renal/nonrenal)				
Blunt trauma	History, variable presentation	Gross/micro	Negative	Renal contusion, etc.
Renal calculi	Severe back and abdominal pain	Gross/micro	Negative	Idiopathic, UTI, calcium, uric acid; IVP indicated
Urethral or meatal injury/foreign body	Frequency, pain; maceration	Gross/micro	Negative	Experimenting, masturbation
Congenital (extraglomerular/ glomerular)				
Hydronephrosis	Abdominal mass	Micro	Positive	Commonly UPJ valve
Polycystic kidney	Large kidney, cystic anomaly	Micro	Positive	Infant, adult
Hemangioma	Variable vascular malformation	Micro	Negative	Rendu-Osler-Weber
Hemoglobinopathy	Hyposthenuria, other signs/symptoms	Micro	Negative	Sickle cell, SC, etc.

Table 41-1. Hematuria and Proteinuria: Etiologic Considerations (*continued*)

Condition	Diagnostic Findings	Hematuria	Proteinuria	Comments
Coagulopathy	Bleeding diathesis	Gross/micro	Negative	Bleeding screen
Hereditary nephritis/ hematuria	Intermittent or persistent; hearing loss	Micro	Negative	Glomerular
Intoxication (extraglomerular)				
Anticoagulants	Nephritis or crystallinuria	Gross/micro	Variable	Temporally related to drug use
Aspirin				
Sulfonamides				
Methicillin				
Neoplasm (extraglomerular)				
Wilm's tumor	Abdominal mass	Gross/micro	Negative	CT, surgical approach
Leukemia	Systemic disease	Micro	Variable	Oncologist

	Glomerular	Extra glomerular or nonrenal
Urine color	Brown, smoky "cola color"	Red, pink, or bright red blood
RBC casts	Common	Absent
Blood clots	Absent	Common

Drugs and other agents that cause a red or dark urine include aniline dyes, blackberries, beets, phenolphthalein, phenytoin (Dilantin), pyrvinium (Povan), phenothiazines, phenozopyridine (Pyridium), rifampin, lead, iron, mercury, and urates.

Proteinuria is often orthostatic in origin, occurring in the upright position. It resolves in 50% of children by early adulthood. Evaluation of orthostatic proteinuria requires careful collection and comparison of standing and recumbent urines. The diagnosis is dependent upon the proteinuria being the only abnormal finding, it being of only minimal amount (up to 5 times normal), and the remainder of the history and physical being normal.

Artifactual proteinuria may result from extraneous sources of protein (i.e., vaginal discharge) or inadequate fluid intake. Significant proteinuria is often associated with hematuria or other abnormalities of urinary sediment. The nephrotic range is usually 5–10 times normal (> 3.5 gm/1.73 m^2/24 hr).

Diagnostic Approach

1. *History* must focus on preexisting conditions.
   a. Urine appearance, frequency, and amount.
   b. Family history of renal disease, deafness, hematuria, edema.
   c. Problems with rash, arthralgia, illness, drugs, exposure to tuberculosis, and systemic signs or symptoms such as edema, anorexia, and weight loss.
2. *Physical examination* should concentrate on cardiovascular stability.
   a. Vital signs measurements including blood pressure (orthostatic), pulse, respiration, temperature, weight, and pallor.
   b. Cardiac and respiratory status.
   c. Palpation of bladder, kidney, external genitalia.
3. *Diagnostic work-up* must rapidly determine if hematuria or proteinuria are present.
   a. *Hematuria* can be detected through chemical tests for blood and microscopic examination of the urine specimen.
      (1) Laboratory.
         (a) Urine dipstik tests change color with the oxidation of orthotolidine to cumene hyproperioxide with the catalysis by hemoglobin or myoglobin.
            (i) Oxidizing agents such as povidone-iodine, hexachlorophene, or hypochlorite may cause false positives, as can a markedly alkaline urine.
            (ii) False negatives can result from ascorbic acid.
         (b) Evaluation of the patient with persistent hematuria of a nontraumatic nature is summarized in Table 41-2.
         (c) Traumatic hematuria, documented by microscopic examination, requires evaluation to define the injury. Myoglobinuria may be a cause of a positive dipstik.
      (2) Radiology evaluation may include:
         (a) Abdominal flat plate to exclude bony and other pathology.
         (b) Retrograde urethrogram if there is blood at the meatus, significant scrotal or perineal hematoma, or obvious urethral trauma.
         (c) Cystogram for bladder injury, pelvic fracture, inadequate urine production, or gross hematuria.
         (d) Excretory urography (IVP) with hematuria, penetrating injury to flank, back, or abdomen, possibly involving the GU tract, flank or costovertebral angle (CVA) tenderness, or unexplained ileus. Some clinicians have suggested that following blunt trauma if there is less than 50 RBC/HPF, the patient can generally be observed without performing an IVP if there are no

other findings. With worrisome findings or greater than 50 RBC/HPF, an IVP should generally be done.

(e) Other studies may include a CT scan, isotopic renal scanning, or arteriography.

b. *Proteinuria* is similarly measured by dipstik, with close correlation between the strip and quanitative determination. However, 50% of "trace" proteinuria have normal protein excretion quantitatively. False positive results occur with highly alkaline urines (pH > 6.5) or contamination with benzalkonium.

(1) Laboratory.

(a) Protein excretion should be determined by 24-hour urine collection and measurement.

(b) Orthostatic proteinuria requires careful collection and comparison of standing and recumbent urines. During a 24-hour collection, separate voids during the night and upon awakening (recumbent position) from the remainder. It requires the proteinuria to be an isolated finding and quantitatively less than 5 times normal.

(c) Evaluation is outlined in Table 41-3.

Alert: Hematuria and proteinuria may be early findings in significant nontraumatic renal disease. Independently, they require an individualized systematic approach to evaluation.

Table 41-2. Diagnostic Work-up for Hematuria

1. History: illness, rashes, arthralgia, growth pattern, TB exposure, family history of renal failure, deafness, hematuria
2. Physical examination: blood pressure, cardiac and pulmonary examination; palpation of bladder and kidneys
3. Urinalysis: microscopic for free RBCs and RBC casts; dipstik to estimate amount of hematuria and proteinuria; specific gravity to assess renal concentrating ability
4. Urine culture
5. Ancillary data
   a. Renal function: BUN, creatinine, 24 hr creatinine clearance and protein excretion
   b. Etiology: streptozyme, ANA, immunoglobulins, complement (CH_{50}, C_3, C_4)
6. Assessment of above tests
   a. *If Normal*: repeat urinalysis three times and if blood persistent, do an IVP
   b. *If Abnormal*: nephrology consult for probable biopsy with concordant evaluation of etiology including TB, VDRL, biopsy

Table 41-3. Diagnostic Work-up for Proteinuria

1. History: exercise, fever, illness, edema, urine output, weight gain
2. Physical examination: blood pressure, edema
3. Urinalysis: dipstik and 24-hour urine for protein, including evaluation for orthostatic changes
4. Assessment of urinalysis
   a. *If trace* to 1+ Protein, recheck at later visit
   b. *If* ≥ 2+ *or persistent:*
      (1) Collect 24-hour urine for creatinine clearance and total protein (> 200 mg/24 hr: pathologic; > 3.5 gm/1.73 m^2/24 hr: nephrotic range)
      (2) BUN, creatinine, total protein, albumin, cholesterol, nephrology consult
      (3) With this evaluation, classify
         (a) Impaired function: ultrasound, IVP, consider biopsy
         (b) Nephrotic range, typical course, age 1–6 yr: protocol for supposed nil disease including steroids
         (c) Nephrotic range and < 1 yr or > 6 yr, glomerulonephritis, or decreasing function: consider biopsy with IVP

Bibliography

Dodge WF, West EF, Smith FH, et al.: Proteinuria and hematuria in school children: epidemiology and early natural history. J Pediatr 88:327, 1976.

Northway J: Hematuria in children. J Pediatr 78:381, 1971.

42 Testicular Pain

Testicular pain is uncommon in the pediatric population but requires assessment of potential emergent conditions.

Etiologic Considerations

Testicular, scrotal, and groin swelling or pain present an array of differential considerations that may be difficult to clinically distinguish (Table 42-1).

Nontender scrotal swelling with an enlarged testicle may be associated with a testicular tumor or antenatal testicular torsion. If the testicle is normal and there is scrotal swelling, a varicocele, spermatocele, hydrocele, incarcerated hernia, Henoch-Schonlein purpura, insect bite, or generalized edema should be considered.

A nontender testicle with a *painful scrotal swelling* may be due to an incarcerated hernia or torsion of the appendix testicle. In addition, torsion of the spermatic cord, Henoch-Schonlein purpura, and tumor must be considered. If the testis is tender, testicular torsion, trauma, and epididymitis/orchitis may be causative.

Diagnostic Approach

1. *History* should focus on the nature of the pain and predisposing conditions.
   - **a.** Preexisting trauma, viral infection (mumps), systemic signs or symptoms.
   - **b.** Rapidity of onset of swelling. Whether pain is sharp or dull, location, radiation, positions that worsen, as well as response to warmth, coolness, and position.
2. *Physical examination.*
   - **a.** Careful examination of scrotum, testicle, epididymis, hernia, prostate, and abdomen.
   - **b.** Doppler examination for testicular blood flow.
3. *Diagnostic work-up.*
   - **a.** Laboratory.
     - **(1)** Urinalysis and culture (epididymitis may have white blood cells).
     - **(2)** Urethral discharge and culture.
   - **b.** Radiologic evaluation should be a technetium scan if torsion considered.

Alert: Painful testicular swelling should focus on excluding testicular torsion before assuming it is infectious in origin.

Bibliography

Haynes BE and Bessen HA: Diagnosis of testicular torsion. JAMA 249:2522, 1983.

May DC, Lesh P, Lewis S, et al.: Evaluation of acute scrotum pain with testicular scanning. Ann Emerg Med 14:696, 1985.

Table 42-1. Testicular Pain: Etiologic Considerations

Condition	Diagnostic Findings	Comments
Testicular torsion	Acute onset of pain; unilateral, tender testicle, horizontal lie; abdominal pain; urine normal; technetium scan, decreased activity; Doppler, decreased	May follow trauma; occurs in sleep; immediate consult
Trauma (Hematocele)	Sudden pain and swelling of testicle; follows trauma; hematoma; urine normal; technetium scan, Doppler variable	Variable types of trauma
Epididymitis/ orchitis	Gradual onset; tender diffuse epididymis or testicle; variable prostatic tenderness; urine, pyuria; technetium scan, increased activity; Doppler, normal; if discharge, may have PMNs on smear	Uncommon before puberty; may be associated with trauma, lifting, exercise; viral: infectious orchitis
Neoplasm	Gradual onset; large, hard, irregular painless testicle; urine and Doppler normal, technetium variably diagnostic	Surgical biopsy

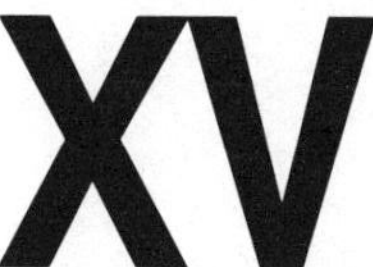

XV Respiratory Problems

43 Apnea

Apnea occurs with a respiratory pause of more than 20 seconds or less than 20 seconds if there is associated bradycardia, cyanosis, pallor, or limping. It must be distinguished from normal breathing irregularities during sleep, which may consist of alternating periods of regular breathing and respiratory pauses of 10 seconds, without color changes, in up to 3% of sleep time. Normal newborns, and particularly premature infants, may demonstrate apneic episodes associated with pauses over 2 seconds.

Respiration is controlled in the pons and medulla, the response to hypoxia differing in newborns and older patients. Hypoxemia normally increases respiratory rate; in newborns however, a brief increase is quickly followed by depression of the respiratory drive and subsequent apnea. Exogenous factors in addition to hypoxia may depress respirations.

Central apnea is marked by an absence of respiratory effort due to lack of activation of the musculature that produces air flow. Although common in premature children, the incidence is inversely proportional to gestation age.

Obstructive apnea occurs when airflow ceases even though respiratory effort with chest and abdominal breathing continues. Airway constriction and dilation combined with the anatomical size of the airway have an impact on air flow.

Etiologic Considerations

1. Infants may suffer apnea as a nonspecific response to a variety of clinical conditions (Table 43-1). Although near-SIDS is perhaps most common, as well as most frightening, other concerns must include seizures, trauma, breath-holding, infection, metabolic derangements, and gastroesophageal reflux or feeding.

   Patients with seizures lose consciousness and then become cyanotic; those with breath-holding spells become cyanotic and then become unconscious. Seizures may follow a breath-holding spell.
2. Older children may suffer obstructive apnea, often during sleep. Restless sleep patterns and apnea may result from tonsillar and adenoidal hypertrophy.

Diagnostic Approach

1. *History* is essential in the evaluation of the child, focusing on substantiating the episode, demonstrating its associated problems, and drawing conclusions about potential etiologies.
   a. Determine the nature of sleep, feeding, reflux, and chalasia. Sleep pattern should be defined with respect to snoring, fitfulness, restlessness, and hypersomnolence.
   b. Define intercurrent illness including viral or bacterial disease, mental status, history of seizures, and metabolic abnormality.
   c. Prenatal and neonatal history.
   d. Family history of apnea, SIDS, respiratory or cardiac problems.
   e. Nature of the episode.

Table 43-1. Apnea: Etiologic Considerations

	Apnea in the Infant	Obstructive Apnea
Infection	Viral: respiratory syncytial (RSV), other Bacterial: pertussis, botulism Meningitis/encephalitis	Tonsillitis, pharyngitis (Chap. 17) Laryngospasm Epiglottitis/croup
Metabolic	Hypoglycemia Hyponatremia Hypocalcemia Encephalopathy	Hypothyroidism Cushing's disease Obesity: Pickwickian Prader Willi
Trauma	Concussion or more severe head injury	Neck injury Foreign body
Congenital	Vascular ring Congenital heart disease Dysrhythmia	Pierre-Robin
Miscellaneous	Near-SIDS (p. 278) Gastroesophageal reflux Breath-holding Overdose Anemia	Laryngomalacia Seizure Seizure Tumor Muscular dystropy

(1) Appearance of the child with respect to color, tone (increased with seizures, choking, aspiration; decreased with prolonged seizure, hypoxia), activity, and respirations.
(2) Precipitating events, past medical history, interval since last feeding, intervention required, and so on.
(3) Duration of the event and sequelae.
(4) Response to stimuli.
(5) Pattern of progression.
(6) Ultimately, the issue is how significant was the episode?

2. *Physical examination* is commonly normal without any specific entity that could account for the seizure. Special attention must be given to:
   a. Assurance that the child is stable and intervention begun if needed.
   b. Careful evaluation of cardiac, neurologic, and respiratory systems.
   c. Focused exam searching for underlying condition.
3. *Diagnostic work-up* should consist of a number of steps to assure some consistency of your evaluation; also watch the child carefully.
   a. Laboratory.
      (1) Hematology: CBC.
      (2) Chemistry: electrolytes, BUN, Ca^{++}.
      (3) Oximetry.
      (4) EEG if any question of seizure, altered mental status, or nystagmus associated with episode.
   b. Radiologic studies include consideration of chest x-ray, CT, nuclear medicine, and barium swallow.
   c. Therapeutic trials may include a variety of approaches that are both diagnostic and therapeutic, all of which require tremendous support.
      (1) Apnea monitors are often sent home with children that have reported apnea. Its benefits versus its risks are not yet established.
      (2) Initiating low dose theophylline (5 mg/kg/24 hr).
      (3) Evaluation for tonsillectomy and adenoidectomy in the older, at-risk child.

Alert: Evidence or suspicion of apnea requires observation and diagnostic evaluation usually in an inpatient setting.

Bibliography

Mathew OP: Maintenance of upper airway patency. J Pediatr 106:863, 1985.

National Institutes of Health: Consensus development conference on infantile apnea and home monitoring – 1986. Pediatrics 79:292, 1987.

Weinstein SL and Steinschneider A: Prolonged infantile apnea: diagnostic and therapeutic dilemma. J Respir Dis 1:76, 1981.

44 Cough

Coughing follows forceful expiration and opening of a closed glottis. An initial inspiration is followed by closure of the glottis. The intrathoracic pressure increases with sudden opening of the glottis and release of intrathoracic air with contraction of diaphragm, chest and abdominal wall, and pelvic floor musculature. The cough reflex may be initiated voluntarily or by a medullary cough center. Excitatory cough receptors are located throughout the respiratory tract (nose, ear, sinus, pharynx, larynx, trachea, bronchi, and bronchioles). Coughing generally provides a protective mechanism, serving to dislodge and remove secretions, exudates, and foreign bodies; it may on occasion interfere with respiratory effort, normal activity, or have associated vomiting.

Coughing is primarily an indication of respiratory disease. Stimuli of the reflex are inflammatory, mechanical from a foreign body or reflux, chemical from ingestion or inhalation, and thermal from hot or cold injuries. However, the cough reflex is minimal in young infants as well as individuals with significant weakness or paralysis; the absence of a cough in these age groups can be problematic.

(See also p. 251.)

Etiologic Considerations

The predominant cause of coughing in children is upper respiratory tract infections. Other causes are age dependent.

Infants experience structural abnormalities of the airway, gastroesophageal reflux, tracheoesophageal fistula, vascular rings, and other anomalies.

Toddlers may have a foreign body, irritation of the airway (especially passive smoking), or asthma.

Children often have asthma, sinusitis, or chronic rhinitis.

Adolescents commonly have a cough caused by smoking or psychogenic factors. A chronic cough may be the clinical presentation of reactive airway disease; other entities to consider include a foreign body, an unusual infection, or a congenital anomaly. On rare occasions, an extrinsic mass effect from a retropharyngeal abscess, mediastinal tumor, or lymph node may cause coughing.

The type or pattern of the cough may be useful in defining differential entities. Coughs that *worsen at night* are usually caused by posterior nasal drips from allergy or upper respiratory infection, while coughs that *improve during sleep* are typically psychogenic in origin. *Productive* coughs imply that there is lower airway, parenchymal infection; *purulent* sputum is associated with bacterial pneumonia, lung abscess, bronchiectasis, and cystic fibrosis. Staccato paroxysmal coughs accompany pertussis or chlamydia infections. A barking or brassy cough and voice change are due to laryngotracheal disease (Table 44-1).

Table 44-1. Cough: Etiologic Considerations

Condition	Diagnostic Findings	Ancillary data	Comments
Infection/Inflammation			
Upper respiratory infection (URI)	Acute onset with variable course; nonproductive; rhinorrhea, fever, pharyngitis, cough worse when lying down due to posterior nasal drip	Throat culture, if indicated	Self-limited; symptomatic treatment
Pneumonia (Chap. 46)	Variable; fever, tachypnea, productive cough, pleuritic pain, hemoptysis	Chest x-ray film; CBC, ABG, if needed	Viral, bacterial, mycoplasma, fungal, TB, chlamydia; antibiotics, if needed
Sinusitis	Nasal discharge, asymmetrical discomfort, congestion, headache	Sinus films	Decongestants, antibiotics, drainage
Bronchiolitis	Wheezing, tachypnea, nonproductive cough, fever, variable cyanosis, apnea	Chest x-ray film; ABG/oximetry, if needed	Viral (RSV); support, hydrate, bronchodilators
Pertussis (whooping cough)	Catarrhal phase followed by paroxysmal cough with cyanosis, vomiting; prolonged cough	Chest x-ray; lymphocytosis with WBC; fluorescent antibody positive	Support; erythromycin
Measles (Chap. 13)	Coryza, conjunctivitis, cough with generalized morbilliform rash; fever, toxic; rare encephalitis, pneumonia	Chest x-ray film if toxic	Support; treat secondary infections
Allergic			
Asthma	Wheezing, tachypnea, variable respiratory distress and cyanosis; nonproductive cough may be only symptom	Chest x-ray film if severe or unresponsive; ABG/oximetry	Oxygen, bronchodilators
Trauma			
Foreign body	If tracheal, partial or total obstruction; if bronchial, nonproductive cough, asymmetrical wheezing	Chest x-ray film (inspiratory and expiratory); direct visualization	Remove by thrust or bronchoscopy

Table 44-1. Cough: Etiologic Considerations (*continued*)

Condition	Diagnostic Findings	Ancillary Data	Comments
Congenital			
Cystic fibrosis	Chronic productive cough, failure to thrive, recurrent pulmonary infection, abnormal stools	Chest x-ray films, ABG, pulmonary function, positive sweat test	Postural drainage; antibiotics, dietary supplement
Tracheoesophageal fistula	Variable cough with feeding; poor weight gain, vomiting	Chest x-ray film, barium swallow	Support, surgery
Diaphragmatic hernia	Acute onset cyanosis as newborn with poor feeding, vomiting, respiratory distress	Chest x-ray film, barium swallow	Support, surgery
Vascular			
Congestive heart failure	Tachypnea, tachycardia, murmur, rales, wheezing cyanosis, cadiomegaly, productive cough	Chest x-ray film; ABG, ECG	Diuretics, digitalis, evaluate cause
Intoxication			
Hydrocarbon ingestion and other chemical inhalations	Initially asymptomatic, then chemical pneumonitis	Chest x-ray film	Postural drainage
Neoplasm			
Pulmonary or mediastinal	Insidious onset, variable cough, hemoptysis, weight loss; chronically ill	Chest x-ray film; nuclear scan, biopsy	Oncologic evaluation

Diagnostic Approach

1. *History* should determine the nature of the cough.
   a. Duration, frequency, timing, quality, and productivity (type of material produced) of the cough. Inciting and ameliorating conditions should be defined.
   b. Associated signs and symptoms such as fever, shortness of breath, respiratory compromise, decreased exercise tolerance, wheezing, allergies, and growth pattern.
   c. Family history should be obtained, focusing particularly on asthma, smoking habits, tuberculosis, cystic fibrosis, and any chronic pulmonary diseases.
   d. Environmental concerns including passive smoking and chemical inhalation should be reviewed.
   e. *Hemoptysis* or coughing up blood, often mixed with sputum (appearing red and frothy), is an unusual pediatric condition that may be associated with a number of specific clinical entities:
      (1) Infection: pneumonia (group A streptococci, tuberculosis), pertussis, pulmonary abscess, bronchiectasis (cystic fibrosis), and viral infections.
      (2) Allergic: following acute asthmatic attack.
      (3) Trauma: foreign body.
      (4) Vascular: pulmonary hypertension, mitral stenosis, pulmonary embolism, pulmonary stenosis.
      (5) Neoplasm: mediastinal or pulmonary.
      (6) Bleeding diathesis.
      (7) Idiopathic pulmonary hemosiderosis.
2. *Physical examination* is often normal, but specific attention must be directed toward evidence of respiratory compromise and the adequacy of airway and ventilation.
   a. Color, respiratory rate, pattern, effort, retractions, and flaring should all be assessed. Careful evaluation of the level of respiratory tract involvement must define wheezing, rhonchi, rales, altered breath sounds, and symmetry.
   b. Evidence of an acute infection may exist, including fever, adenopathy, productive cough, rhinorrhea, or rash.
   c. Allergic disease may be evaluated by looking for eczema, boggy nasal mucosa, clear rhinorrhea, hypertrophic lymphoid follicles, and allergic shiners.
3. *Diagnostic work-up* is rarely required unless the cough is clearly associated with systemic disease, is prolonged, or the history or physical examination are particularly worrisome. Oximetry may be useful.
   a. Laboratory evaluation may include:
      (1) A CBC may provide evidence of infection, atopy (eosinophilia), or polycythemia and may be useful in monitoring infection.
      (2) Blood cultures are indicated in febrile toxic patients with a course consistent with a bacterial infection. Children with productive coughs who can expectorate may benefit from a microscopic examination of the sputum, including appearance, cellular composition, Gram's stain, and culture.
      (3) Pulmonary function testing may be useful in children with restrictive or obstructive disease who are chronically ill or unresponsive to acute management. Bronchoscopy may contribute to evaluation for foreign body, atelectasis, aberrant anatomy, or unusual parenchymal disease. Specific additional studies that may be considered include sweat testing, immunoglobulin levels, alpha-1-antitrypsin levels, nasal smear for eosinophils, and skin testing. A response to nebulization or metered dose inhaler (MDI) therapy may be useful in confirming reactive airway disease.
      (4) Bronchoscopy should be considered as an additional therapeutic and diagnostic maneuver.
   b. Radiologic assessment may include a chest x-ray study, including inspiratory and expiratory studies if a foreign body is suspected. Sinus, neck, and barium swallow examinations may be considered in specific circumstances.

c. Therapeutic trials may be instigated.

(1) Bronchodilators, especially beta 2 agonist agents such as albuterol, may be useful in defining whether there is a reactive component.

(2) In the face of a persistent cough and a noncontributory evaluation, empirical trials of antibiotics, or decongestants prior to sleep may be initiated as part of the evaluation to exclude posterior nasal drip, depending upon the nature of the presentation of the cough.

Alert: Although coughing is usually benign, association with lower respiratory tract infection or other conditions must be excluded. Respiratory distress must also be excluded.

Bibliography

Denny F: Acute respiratory infections in children: etiology and epidemiology. Pediatr Rev 9:135, 1987.

Hannaway PJ and Hopper DK: Cough variant asthma in children. JAMA 247:206, 1982.

Mellis CM: Evaluation and treatment of chronic cough in children. Pediatr Clin North Am 26:553, 1979.

45 Cyanosis

Decreased oxygenation of blood produces cyanosis. For it to be clinically evident, there must be at least 5 g of reduced Hgb/dl, usually associated with an oxyhemoglobin saturation of 85% or less. Because of the increased affinity of fetal hemoglobin for oxygen, the infant may have hypoxia without cyanosis. Desaturation is most evident in areas of the epidermis that are relatively thin, where pigment is minimal and capillaries abundant, such as the tips of the fingers and toes, under the nail beds, and in the buccal mucosa (Table 45-1).

Etiologic Considerations

1. *Central cyanosis* is reflected clinically in the tongue, mucosal membranes, and peripheral skin. Physiologic conditions producing cyanosis may include:
   - **a.** Decreased pulmonary and alveolar ventilation with impaired oxygen intake. This responds moderately to administration of oxygen.
   - **b.** Decreased pulmonary perfusion with marked pulmonary shunting of blood responding minimally, if at all, to administration of 100% oxygen.
   - **c.** Abnormal hemoglobin. Methemoglobin produces cyanosis when it exceeds 15% of the total hemoglobin.
2. *Peripheral cyanosis* commonly has a vascular etiology leading to a bluish discoloration of the skin in the absence of central cyanosis.
   - **a.** Vascular instability may accompany sepsis. In newborns it may also occur with temperature changes or metabolic abnormalities.
   - **b.** Capillary stasis or venous pooling.
   - **c.** Raynaud's phenomenon.
   - **d.** Hematologic.
     - **(1)** Polycythemia due to congenital heart disease, chronic hypoxia, or maternal-fetal or twin-twin transfusion.
     - **(2)** Hyperviscosity.
   - **e.** Harlequin color changes are benign, accompanied by half of the body becoming pale or acutely reddened for a few minutes.

Diagnostic Approach

1. *History* should focus on potential contributory conditions.
   - **a.** History of congenital heart, lung, or GI disease, family history of cardiac or pulmonary disease, or perinatal problems.
   - **b.** Pattern of onset of cyanosis and respiratory distress. Factors that make worse or reduce.
   - **c.** Recent onset of fever, infection, shortness of breath.
   - **d.** Traumatic episode or foreign body.
   - **e.** Ingestion of well water or exposure to carbon monoxide.
   - **f.** Behavioral or neurological abnormalities or concerns.

Table 45-1. Cyanosis: Etiologic Considerations

Condition	Mechanism/ Response to 100% O_2	Ancillary Data
Vascular – Cardiac		
Congenital heart disease		
↓ pulmonary blood flow	↓ perfusion/shunting Little response	ABG: ↓ PaO_2, ↓ ↑ pH CXR: ↓ PBF, ↑ heart (right-left shunt) Hypoglycemia
↑ pulmonary blood flow	↑ perfusion/shunting Little response	ABG: ↓ PaO_2, ↑ ↓ pH CXR: ↑ PBF, ↑ heart (right-left shunt) Hypoglycemia
Congestive heart failure (CHF)	↓ alveolar ventilation and perfusion Moderate response	ABG: ↓ PaO_2, ↓ pH, ↑ ↓ $PaCO_2$ CXR: ↑ PBF, pulmonary edema, ↑ heart
Pulmonary edema	↓ alveolar ventilation Moderate response	ABG: ↓ PaO_2, ↓ ↑ pH, ↑ $PaCO_2$ CXR: interstitial edema
Shock (Chap. 3)	↓ perfusion Good response	ABG: ↓ PaO_2, ↓ pH, ↑ ↓ $PaCO_2$
Vascular – Pulmonary		
Pulmonary hemorrhage Pulmonary embolism Persistent fetal newborn circulation Pulmonary AV fistula Pulmonary hypertension	↓ alveolar perfusion Moderate response	ABG: ↓ PaO_2, ↑ ↓ pH, ↑ ↓ $PaCO_2$ CXR: right to left shunt
Vascular ring	↓ ventilation Good response	ABG: ↓ PaO_2, ↑ $PaCO_2$ CXR: hyperexpansion Barium swallow/ bronchoscopy
Vascular – CNS hemorrhage		
Subdural Intracranial	↓ ventilation Moderate response	ABG: ↓ PaO_2, ↑ $PaCO_2$ CT scan: diagnostic
Infection/Inflammation		
Upper airway disease Croup Epiglottitis	↓ ventilation Good response	ABG: ↓ PaO_2, ↓ ↑ pH, ↑ $PaCO_2$
Lower airway disease Pneumonia Asthma Bronchiolitis Atelectasis Aspiration Hyaline membrane disease Cystic fibrosis	↓ alveolar ventilation and perfusion Moderate response	ABG: ↓ PaO_2, ↓ pH, ↑ $PaCO_2$ CXR: diagnostic
Meningitis (Chap. 32) Sepsis	↓ perfusion and ventilation Good response	ABG: ↓ PaO_2, ↓ pH, ↓ ↑ $PaCO_2$

Table 45-1. *(continued)*

Condition	Mechanism/ Response to 100% O_2	Ancillary Data
Trauma		
Foreign body Pneumothorax	↓ perfusion and ventilation Good response	ABG: ↓ PaO_2, ↓ pH, ↑ $PaCO_2$
Congenital		
Hereditary hemoglobinemia	Methemoglobinemia No response	Methemoglobin high
Diaphragmatic hernia Macroglossia Tracheolaryngomalacia	↓ ventilation Good response	ABG: ↓ PaO_2, ↓ ↑ pH, ↑ $PaCO_2$ CXR/lateral neck: diagnostic
Intoxication		
Nitrates, nitrites, aniline dyes, sulfonamides	Methemoglobinemia No response	Methemoglobin high
Carbon monoxide	Displacement O_2 by CO Good response	Carboxyhemoglobin level
Other		
Breath holding	↓ ventilation Moderate response	ABG: ↓ PaO_2, ↑ $PaCO_2$ Self-limited
Seizure (Chap. 36)	↓ ventilation Good response	ABG: ↓ PaO_2, ↓ pH, ↑ $PaCO_2$

2. *Physical examination* should focus on assessing cardiovascular stability, defining the etiologic condition, and making certain that the cyanosis is central and not peripheral.

a. Vital signs and adequacy of airway, ventilation, and circulation.

b. Cardiovascular exam evaluating for murmurs, failure, edema, and dysrhythmias.

c. Pulmonary evaluation to assess underlying acquired or congenital conditions.

d. Mental status and CNS assessment.

3. *Diagnostic work-up.*

a. Laboratory.

(1) Analysis of the ABG (and oximetry monitoring).

(2) Hematocrit and when appropriate, a methemoglobin level. Methemoglobin is elevated when blood turns a chocolate color when exposed to the air.

(3) Chest x-ray film (CXR) is commonly indicated on all patients.

(4) When indicated, an ECG is also appropriate. Specific studies, such as a barium swallow, bronchoscopy, and CT scan, should be obtained to exclude specific entities.

b. Therapeutic trial.

The response to 100% oxygen should be measured by comparing the ABG (or oximetry) in room air and during the administration of high flow (100%) oxygen. This assists in differentiating primary cardiac disease, which does not respond due to major shunting, from pulmonary disease, which is primarily due to ventilation deficits. Examples of changes with various conditions may be depicted as follows:

	Pulmonary disease (ventilation)		Heart disease (perfusion)	
	Room air	100% O_2	Room air	100% O_2
Color	Blue	Pinker	Blue	Blue
PaO_2 (mmHg) (average range: 60–250)	35	120	35 or less	Little change
Oxygen Saturation	60%	90%	60%	65%

Alert: Cyanosis requires immediate treatment and diagnostic evaluation.

Bibliography

Engle MA: Cyanotic congenital heart disease. Am J Cardiol 37:283, 1976.

Keith JD, Rowe RD, Vlad P (ed): *Heart Disease in Infancy and Children, 3rd ed*. New York: Macmillan Pub., 1978.

46 Respiratory Distress (Dyspnea)

Respiratory distress is a common life-threatening presentation resulting from upper or lower tract pulmonary disease.

Etiologic Considerations

Differentiating upper and lower disease is of primary importance, allowing the clinician to narrow the focus upon these common entities that produce respiratory problems in children (Figure 46-1).

Upper airway disease	**Lower airway disease**
Croup	Bronchiolitis
Epiglottitis	Asthma
Foreign body	Pneumonia
Bacterial tracheitis	Foreign body

Stridor is the major complaint with significant upper airway disease. Inspiratory stridor is usually supraglottic, while expiratory stridor emanates from the trachea. Patients with inspiratory and expiratory stridor or expiratory stridor alone usually have more significant obstructions. Supraglottic stridor is usually quiet and may be associated with a muffled voice, dysphagia, and a preference to sit, while subglottic lesions cause stridor, often with a hoarse voice, barky cough, and may cause facial edema. The diagnostic entities to consider include:

1. Supraglottic: croup (virus), epiglottitis *(H. influenzae)*, other bacterial infections (group A streptococcus, *Staphylococcus aureus*, oral anaerobes *[Peptococcus, Bacteroides, cornyebacterium diphtheriae]*).
2. Infra(sub)glottic (laryngitis, laryngotracheitis, laryngotracheobronchitis): viral infection, *Mycoplasma pneumoniae*, and bacterial infections. *Bacterial tracheitis* is a secondary infection involving an inflamed trachea often from an antecedent viral infection. It is commonly due to *Staphylococcus aureus* or *H. influenzae* with accumulation of pus in the trachea causing a thick plug and ultimately leading to obstruction. It is often associated with pneumonia and clinically presents as a "croup-like" syndrome with toxicity and rapid progression.

Lower airway disease consists of a diverse group of entities that affect the ability to ventilate the lungs or perfuse the pulmonary capillaries. It is *not* commonly associated with stridor. The most common causes of lower airway disease are pneumonia and asthma. Pulmonary pathology is often associated with exertional dyspnea, while cardiac conditions often cause orthopnea and paroxysmal nocturnal dyspnea.

Common causes of respiratory distress in *children under 2 years of age* include pneumonia, asthma, croup, congenital heart disease, foreign body aspiration, congenital anomalies of the airway (tracheal web, cysts, lobar emphysema), and nasopharyngeal obstruction (large tonsils and adenoids). *Older children* more frequently have asthma, poisoning, drowning, trauma, cystic fibrosis, peripheral neuritis, or encephalitis as the underlying disease.

In addition to the more common entities associated with primary lung disease, other causes of apparent dyspnea include increased oxygen demand (increased activity, fever,

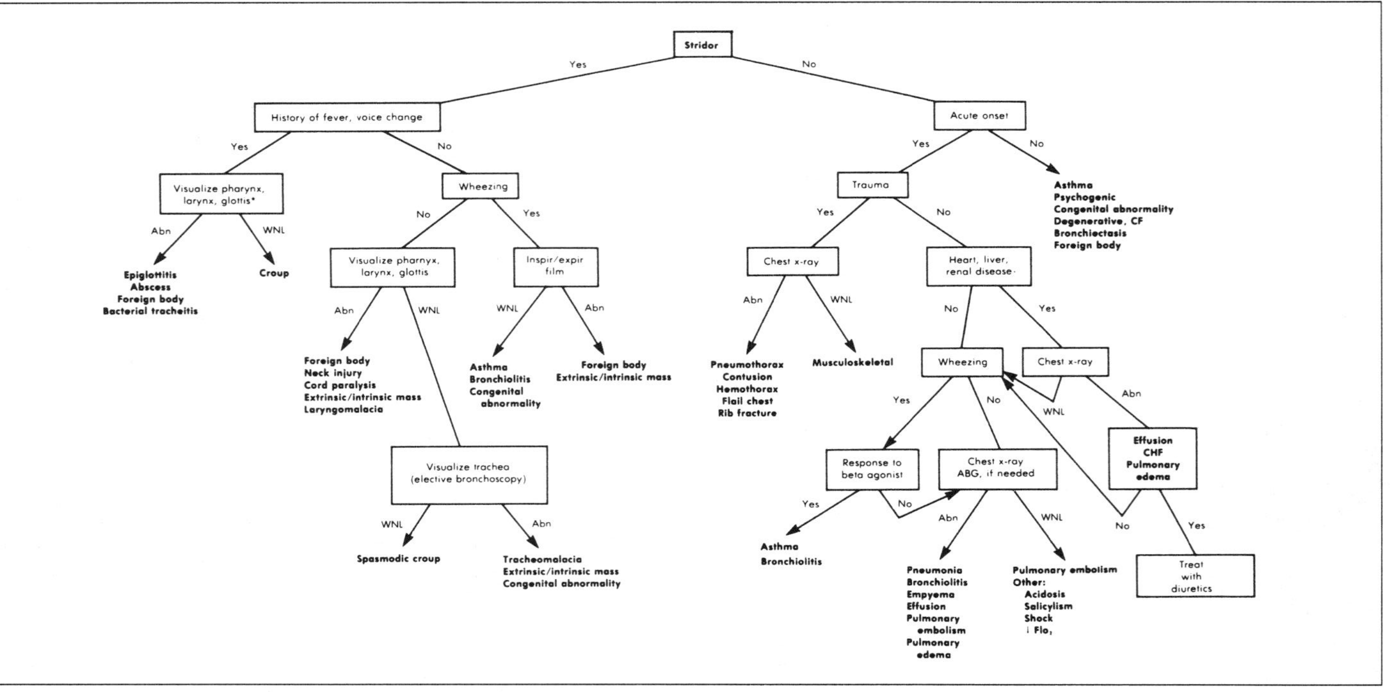

Figure 46-1. Respiratory distress. *Do not visualize without immediate capability of airway intervention. If epiglottitis is suspected, procedure should be performed in operating room. (Reproduced by permission from Barkin RM and Rosen P: *Emergency Pediatrics: A Guide to Ambulatory Care*, (3rd ed.) St. Louis: C. V. Mosby Co 1990.

hyperthyroidism), deficient oxygen transport (anemia, methemoglobinemia, or shock), tachypnea as compensation for a metabolic acidosis (diabetes mellitus, uremia, drug ingestion), low ambient oxygen, central neurogenic stimulation, or progressive spinal or CNS disease (Table 46-1).

Diagnostic Approach

1. *History* must focus on the presenting problems.
   a. Past medical problems related to respiratory distress, recurrent problems with shortness of breath, cough, pneumonia, retractions, and fever. Exposure to potential chemical or environmental irritants.
   b. Family history of recurrent pulmonary or cardiac disease, infectious exposures, TB, and early death.
   c. Current episode including nature of progression, associated signs and symptoms, cough (productive versus unproductive), fever, chest pain, trauma, and foreign body ingestion. Evidence of retractions, tachypnea, wheezing, stridor, relationship with eating, and so on.
2. *Physical examination* must include evaluation of the respiratory tract and associated problems.
   a. Assess the stability of the airway and ventilatory status. It is essential to know the normal respiratory rate, pulse, and blood pressure on an age-specific basis.
   b. Respiratory status evaluation must also include:
      (1) Air entry and type of breathing.
      (2) Color.
      (3) Retractions.
      (4) Breath sounds.
      (5) Stridor.
   c. Airway integrity and ventilatory status can be rapidly assessed initially by evaluating for the presence of *stridor* or auscultation to determine the adequacy of air movement and whether wheezing, rales, or ronchi are present. Obviously the diagnostic considerations are broadened to include pneumothorax and hemothorax if there is preceding trauma.
3. *Diagnostic work-up* must distinguish the type of underlying condition.
   a. Upper airway obstruction: laboratory evaluation is usually ancillary to direct visualization, particularly in patients with respiratory distress. This must be done with great caution and anticipation, being prepared to support the airway. Specific measures are indicated by specific conditions. In selected circumstances, lateral neck x-ray, bronchoscopy, and other specialized procedures.
   b. Lower airway disease: chest x-ray and ABG (or oximetry) provide initial data. Specific tests for suspected entities must be obtained.

   Alert: Don't make the child worse; avoid upsetting the patient when possible. Never underestimate the degree of distress nor leave the child unattended in the ED or x-ray, for example, until evaluation and initial stabilization are complete.

Bibliography

Royall JA and Levin DL: Acute respiratory distress syndrome in pediatric patients. J Pediatr 112:169, 1988.

Stempel D and Mellon M: Management of severe asthma. Pediatr Clin North Am 31:879, 1984.

Table 46-1. Respiratory Distress: Etiologic Considerations

Upper Airway Conditions			
Condition	Diagnostic Findings	Ancillary Data	Comments
Infection			
Epiglottitis	Febrile, toxic; inspiratory stridor; cyanosis, drooling, sore throat; cherry red epiglottis	Increased WBC; lateral neck x-ray abnormal	*H. influenzae*; visualize cautiously; life-threatening
Croup	Inspiratory stridor, croupy cough, variable respiratory distress; normal epiglottis	Variable WBC; lateral neck x-ray normal	Viral; trial of mist, steroids, racemic epinephrine
Peritonsillar abscess Retropharyngeal/ esophageal abscess	Fever, severe throat pain, drooling, inspiratory stridor, dysphagia, tonsillar enlargement	Increased WBC; lateral neck x-ray	Surgical evaluation, visualization
Bacterial tracheitis	Febrile, toxic; inspiratory stridor; brassy cough	Increased WBC	Fails to respond to croup therapy; life threatening
Diphtheria	Toxic, slight fever, hoarse, pharyngeal membrane	Culture	Immunized, exposed
Trauma			
Foreign body Pharynx, larynx	History; symptoms reflect level obstruction-cyanosis, stridor, wheezing	Inspiratory/expiratory chest x-ray	First aid – back blow, abdomen/chest thrust
Neck injury	Trauma; instability/disruption neck, larynx; stridor	Cervical spine x-ray; laryngoscopy	Stabilize airway
Congenital			
Vascular ring Laryngeal web Small mandible (Pierre Robin)	Chronic inspiratory/expiratory	Laryngoscopy/bronchoscopy	Stabilize

Tracheomalacia Laryngomalacia	Expiratory stridor Inspiratory stridor	Chest x-ray, laryngoscopy	Changes with position; may resolve
Allergic			
Croup, Spasmodic	Rapid onset inspiratory stridor; exposure irritant or sensitizing agent	Response to nebulized racemic epinephrine	
Anaphylaxis Angioneurotic edema	Rapid onset stridor, distress, wheezing; follows exposure to food, insect sting, etc.	Response to nebulized beta agonist	Avoid exposure
Neoplasm			
Neck, tracheal, esophageal	Progression stridor, dysphagia, systemic problems	Direct laryngoscopy, x-ray	
		Lower Airway Disease	
Infection			
Pneumonia	Fever, toxicity, cough, variable chest sounds	CBC, blood culture, chest x-ray, ABG	Assess respiratory status
Bronchiolitis	Tachypnea, nontoxic, variable cyanosis, wheezing	Oximetry, chest x-ray, response to beta agonist	Respiratory syncytial virus (RSV)
Pulmonary embolism	Tachypnea, hemoptysis, chest pain, variable fever	Chest x-ray, ABG, ventilation/ perfusion scan	Predisposing factors
Vascular			
Congestive heart failure	Orthopnea, rales, edema, fatigue, cough	Chest x-ray, ECG, ABG	Acquired or congenital
Pulmonary edema	Tachypnea, rales, cough, orthopnea, wheezing	Chest x-ray, ECG, ABG	Cardiogenic or noncardiogenic

Table 46-1. Respiratory Distress: Etiologic Considerations (*continued*)

Condition	Diagnostic Findings	Ancillary Data	Comments
Trauma			
Foreign body	History, cough, wheezing, unequal breath sounds	Inspiratory/expiratory chest x-ray; bronchoscopy	
Pneumothorax	Tachypnea, chest pain, unequal breath sounds	Chest x-ray	Trauma or spontaneous
Allergic			
Asthma	Tachypnea, wheezing, cough, variable distress	Chest x-ray, ABG, response beta agonist	Oximetry
Anaphylaxis	Tachypnea, wheezing, exposure	Chest x-ray, ABG	Exposure allergen
Congenital			
Cystic fibrosis	Progressive pulmonary findings (pneumonia, hemoptysis, atelectasis); poor growth; malabsorption, rectal prolapse	Chest x-ray, sweat test	Pulmonary functions, consult
Neoplasm	Progressive disease, symptoms	Chest x-ray, CT	

XVI Traumatic Problems

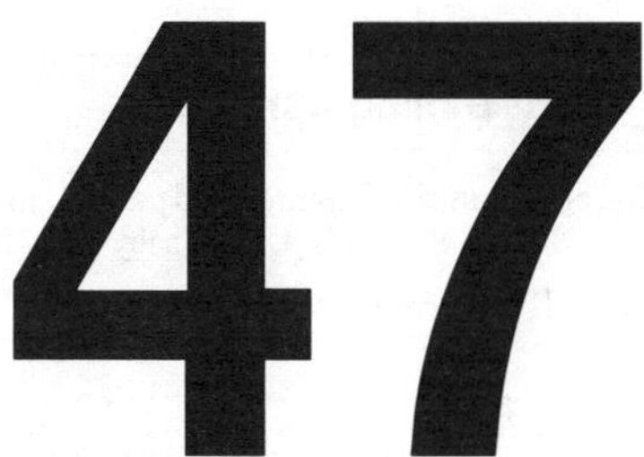

47 The Traumatized Child

Children commonly experience injury from sports, falls, or motor vehicle accidents. The history is usually obvious; the injuries are often hidden. Beyond the principles of immediate assessment and stabilization, the psychologic impact upon the child and family are immense and must be addressed through communication, support, and understanding.

1. *Principles of management* must be consistent, focusing upon an appropriate organization and delegation of responsibilities and a team approach. Aggressive management is essential:
   a. Assume the most serious diagnosis. The most serious and life-threatening condition must be excluded.
   b. Consider the nature and the mechanism of the accident. Children who have experienced an injury caused by a serious accident should be considered significantly injured until proven stable.
   c. Treatment in the unstable patient may need to be based upon clinical findings rather than waiting for laboratory or radiologic confirmation. For example, a tension pneumothorax should be treated on the basis of clinical findings rather than requiring x-ray exam documentation because confirmatory chest x-rays may take too long.

2. *Assessment of priorities* must be done in an orderly fashion.
   a. Assess and stabilize priorities.
      (1) Airway.
      (2) Breathing.
      (3) Circulation.
      (4) Cervical spine (and thoracic and lumbar spine).
   b. Perform a concise, systematic, and thorough examination. Remove all clothing and do not stop looking once you detect one serious injury. More than one may be present.
   c. Frequently reassess the patient. After the initial assessment and stabilization, do a secondary survey looking for other injuries.
      (1) Neurologic.
      (2) Cardiac and thoracic.
      (3) Abdomen.
      (4) Musculoskeletal.
   d. Remember the five tubes approach to resuscitation.
      (1) Two large caliber IV lines.
      (2) NG tube (check for blood).
      (3) Foley bladder tube (check for blood at the urethral meatus; check amount of urine and if there is blood present).
      (4) Tubes of blood for Hct and type and cross-match.
   e. Consider psychologic concerns related to type of injury. The combination of pain, separation, a strange environment, and unfamiliar health professionals places an inordinate stress on patient and family.

Alert: Aggressive management must be the basis for approaching the traumatized child. Stabilization must precede an extensive diagnostic evaluation.

Bibliography

Jorden RC: Evaluation and stabilization of the multiply traumatized patient. In Barkin RM and Rosen P: *Emergency Pediatrics, 3rd ed*. St. Louis: C. V. Mosby Co., 1990.

Moore EE, Eiseman B, and Van Way CW III: *Critical Decisions in Trauma*. St. Louis: C. V. Mosby Co., 1984.

Appendixes

A Vital Signs

Age	Weight (kg)	Heart Rate (avg/min)	Respiratory Rate (avg/min)	Blood Pressure (mean ± 2 SD)	
				Systolic	Diastolic
Premature	1	145	< 40	42 ± 10	21 ± 8
Newborn	1–2	135		50 ± 10	28 ± 8
Newborn	2–3	125		60 ± 10	37 ± 8
1 mo	4	120	24–35	80 ± 16	46 ± 16
6 mo	7	130		89 ± 29	60 ± 10
1 yr	10	125	20–30	96 ± 30	66 ± 25
2–3 yr	12–14	115		99 ± 25	64 ± 25
4–5 yr	16–18	100		99 ± 20	65 ± 20
6–8 yr	20–26	100	12–25	98 ± 15	65 ± 20
10–12 yr	32–42	75		105 ± 15	65 ± 20
> 14 yr	> 50	70	12–18	112 ± 18	65 ± 18

B

Growth Curves

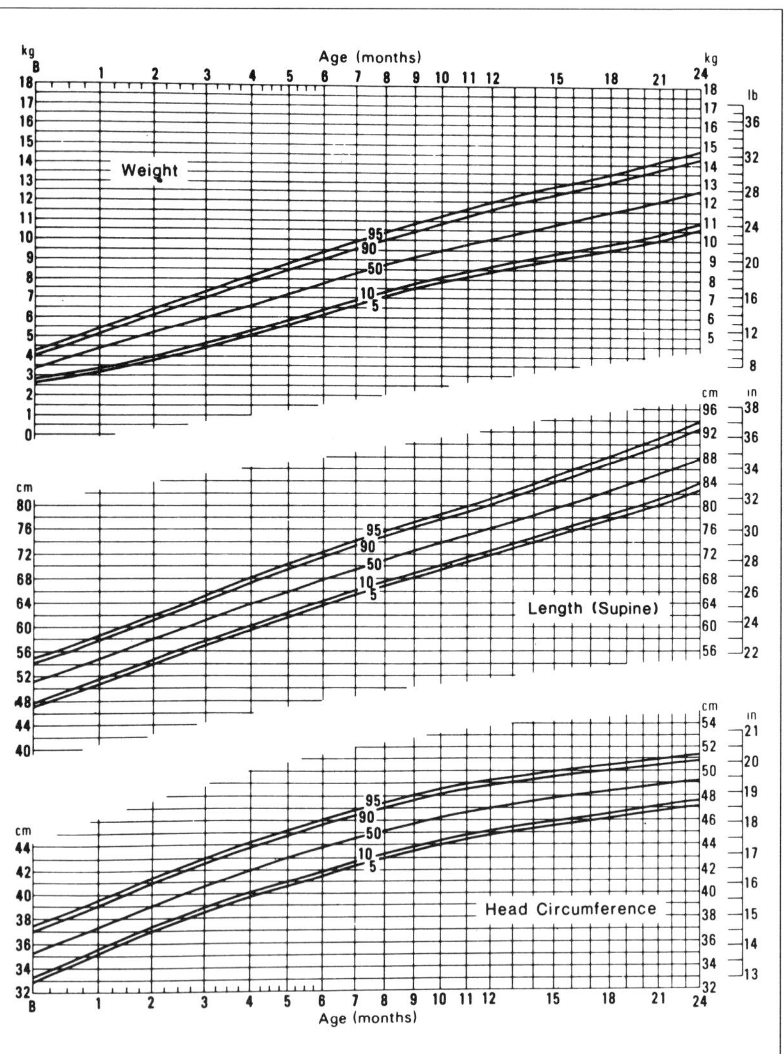

Percentile standards for growth: boys (birth–24 mo). (Modified from National Center for Health Statistics [NCHS] growth charts, 1976.)

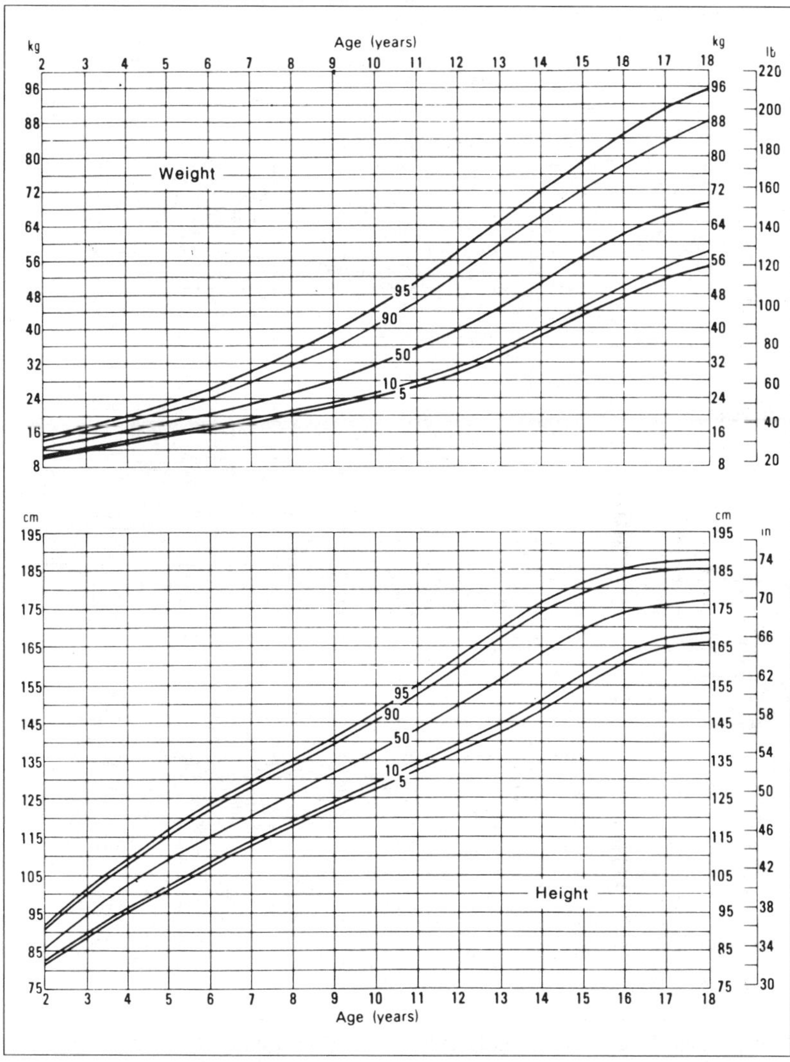

Percentile standards for growth: boys (2–18 yr). (Modified from NCHS growth charts, 1976).

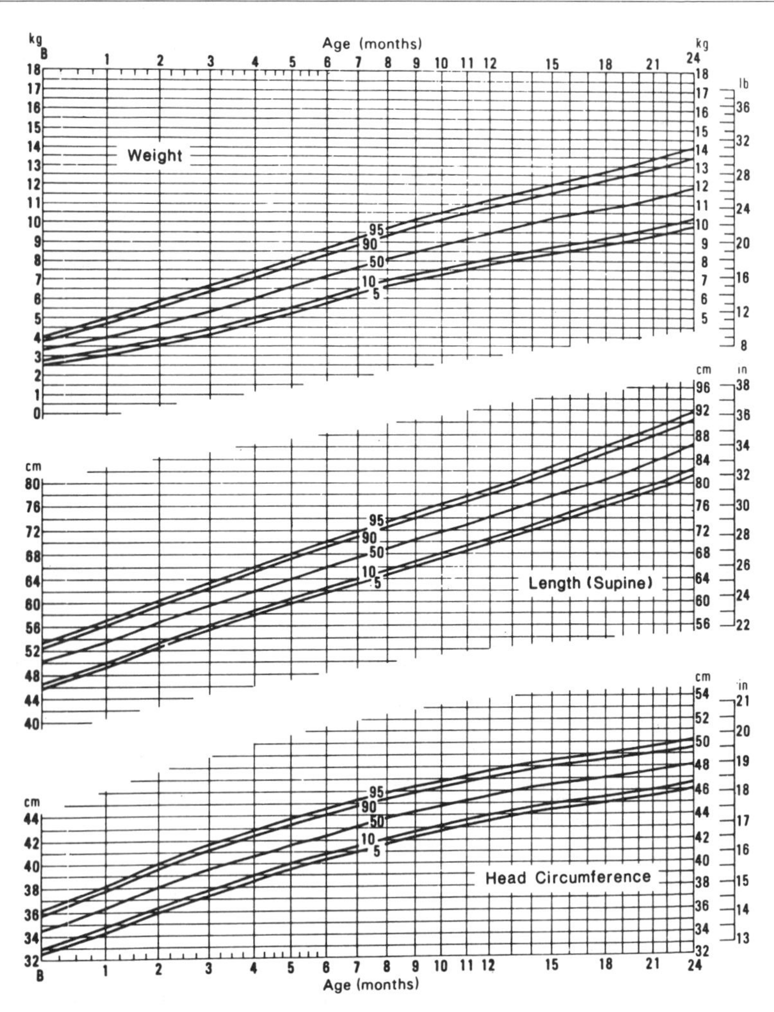

Percentile standards for growth: girls (birth–24 mo). (Modified from NCHS growth charts, 1976.)

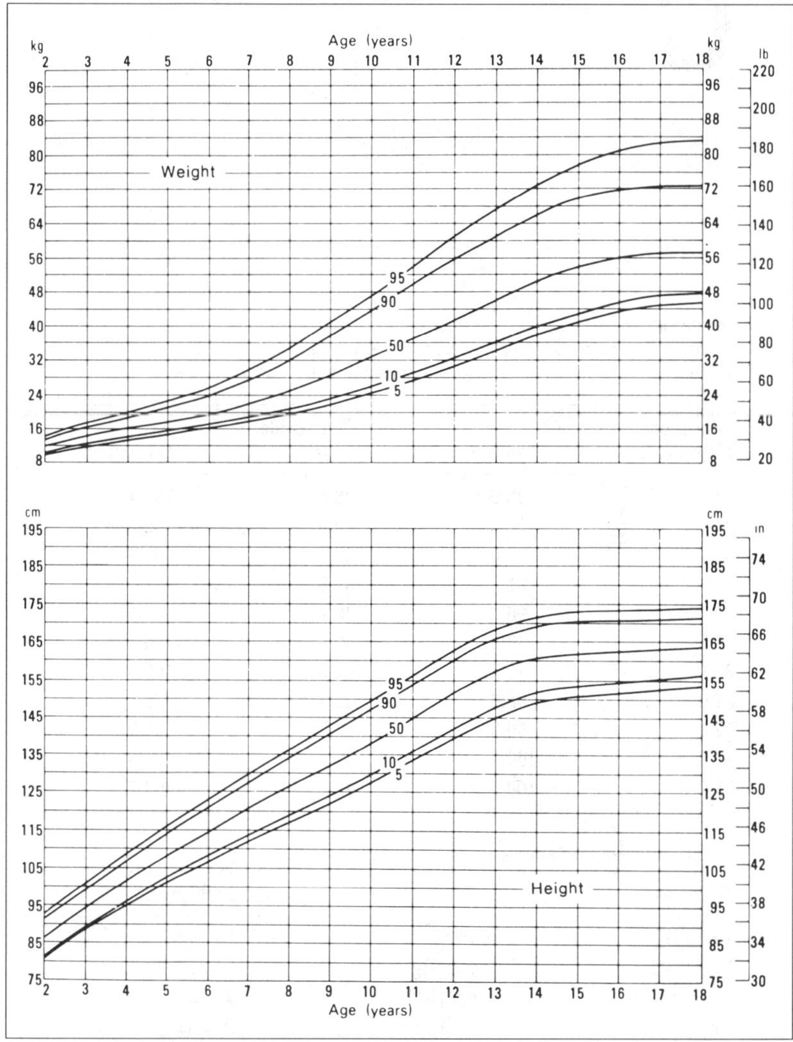

Percentile standards for growth: girls (2–18 yr). (Modified from NCHS growth charts, 1976.) (Reproduced by permission from Barkin RM and Rosen P: *Emergency Pediatrics: A Guide to Ambulatory Care* (3rd ed.), St. Louis: C. V. Mosby Co., 1990.)

C Measurement Conversions

Temperature

To convert centigrade to Fahrenheit: ($9/5$ × temperature) + 32
To convert Fahrenheit to centigrade: (temperature − 32) × $5/9$

Centigrade (Celsius)	Fahrenheit	Centigrade (Celsius)	Fahrenheit
34.2	93.6	38.6	101.4
34.6	94.3	39.0	102.2
35.0	95.0	39.4	102.9
35.4	95.7	39.8	103.6
35.8	96.4	40.2	104.3
36.2	97.1	40.6	105.1
36.6	97.8	41.0	105.8
37.0	98.6	41.4	106.5
37.4	99.3	41.8	107.2
37.8	100.0	42.2	108.0
38.2	100.7	42.6	108.7

Other Conversion Factors

To convert	To	Multiply by
1 mm Hg	PSI	0.0193
1 cm H_2O	mm Hg	0.735
1 mm Hg	cm H_2O	1.259
1 cm	inch	0.3937
1 inch	cm	2.54
1 kg	pound	2.204
1 pound	kg	0.4536
1 Fr size	mm	0.33

Weight Conversion Table (pounds and ounces to grams)

Ounces	0 lb	1 lb	2 lb	3 lb	4 lb	5 lb	6 lb	7 lb	8 lb	9 lb
0		454	907	1361	1814	2268	2722	3175	3629	4082
1	28	482	936	1389	1843	2296	2750	3204	3657	4111
2	57	510	964	1418	1871	2325	2778	3232	3686	4139
3	85	539	992	1446	1899	2353	2807	3260	3714	4168
4	113	567	1020	1474	1928	2382	2835	3289	3742	4196
5	142	595	1049	1503	1956	2410	2863	3317	3771	4224
6	170	624	1077	1531	1984	2438	2892	3345	3799	4253
7	198	652	1106	1559	2013	2467	2920	3374	3827	4281
8	227	680	1134	1588	2041	2495	2948	3402	3855	4309
9	255	709	1162	1616	2070	2523	2977	3430	3884	4338
10	284	737	1191	1644	2098	2552	3005	3459	3912	4366
11	312	765	1219	1673	2126	2580	3034	3487	3940	4394
12	340	794	1247	1701	2155	2608	3062	3516	3969	4423
13	369	822	1276	1729	2183	2637	3090	3544	3997	4451
14	397	850	1304	1758	2211	2665	3119	3572	4026	4479
15	425	879	1332	1786	2240	2693	3147	3601	4054	4508

If patient weighs ≥ 10 lb, the following are used, adding the intermediate value in pounds and ounces to determine the final conversion:

10 lb	4.53 kg	60 lb	27.21 kg	110 lb	49.89 kg	160 lb	72.57 kg
20 lb	9.07 kg	70 lb	31.75 kg	120 lb	54.43 kg	170 lb	77.11 kg
30 lb	13.60 kg	80 lb	36.28 kg	130 lb	58.96 kg	180 lb	81.64 kg
40 lb	18.14 kg	90 lb	40.82 kg	140 lb	63.50 kg	190 lb	86.18 kg
50 lb	22.68 kg	100 lb	45.36 kg	150 lb	68.04 kg	200 lb	90.72 kg

(Reproduced by permission from Barkin RM and Rosen P: *Emergency Pediatrics: A Guide to Ambulatory Care* (3rd ed.), St. Louis: C. V. Mosby Co., 1990.)

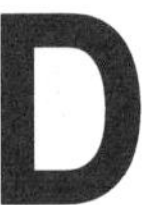

Normal Laboratory Values*

Determinations for:
(S) = Serum
(B) = Whole blood
(P) = Plasma

Acid-base measurements (B)
pH: 7.38–7.42
PaO_2: 65–76 mm Hg
$PaCO_2$: 36–38 mm Hg
Base excess: −2 to +2 mEq/L

Acid Phosphatase (S, P)
Newborns: 7.4–19.4 IU/L
2–13 yr: 6.4–15.2 IU/L
Adult males: 0.5–11 IU/L
Adult females: 0.2–9.5 IU/L

Alanine Aminotransferase (SGPT) (S)
Newborns (1–3 days): 1–25 IU/L
Adult males: 7–46 IU/L
Adult females: 4–35 IU/L

Alkaline Phosphatase (S)

Age	IU/L
Newborns (1–3 days)	95–368
2–24 mo	115–460
2–7 yr	115–460
8–9 yr	115–345
10–11 yr	115–437
12–13 yr	92–403
14–15 yr	78–446
16–18 yr	35–331
Adults	39–137

Ammonia (P)
Newborns: 9–150 μg/dl (53–88 μmol/L); higher in premature and jaundiced infants
Thereafter: 0–60 μg/dl (0–35 μmol/L) when blood is drawn correctly

Amylase (S)
Neonates: undetectable
2–12 mo: levels increase to adult levels
Adults: 28–108 IU/L

*Values may vary with laboratory, technique, determination, underlying conditions, etc.

Aspartate Aminotransferase (SGOT) (S)
Newborns (1–3 days): 16–74 IU/L
Adult males: 8–46 IU/L
Adult females: 7–34 IU/L

Bicarbonate (P)
18–25 mEq/L

Bilirubin (S)
After 1 mo are:
Conjugated: 0–0.3 mg/dl
Unconjugated: 0.1–0.7 mg/dl

Bleeding Time
1–3 min

Calcium (S)
Premature infants: 3.5–4.5 mEq/L
Full-term infants: 4–5 mEq/L
Infants and thereafter: 4.4–5.3 mEq/L

Carboxyhemoglobin (B)
5% of total hemoglobin

Cation-Anion Gap (S, P)
5–15 mEq/L

Chloride (S, P)
96–116 mmol/L

Cholesterol (S, P)
Full-term newborns: 45–167 mg/dl
3 days–1 yr: 69–174 mg/dl
2–14 yr: 120–205 mg/dl
14–19 yr: 120–210 mg/dl

Complement (S)
C3: 96–195 mg/dl
C4: 15–20 mg/dl

Creatinine (S, P)
Values in mg/dl

Age	Males	Females
Newborns (1–3 days)	0.2–1.0	0.2–1.0
1–3 yr	0.2–0.7	0.2–0.6
4–10 yr	0.2–0.9	0.2–0.8
11–17 yr	0.3–1.2	0.3–1.1
>18 yr	0.5–1.3	0.3–1.1

Creatinine Clearance
Newborns: 40–65 ml/min/1.73 m^2 (mean, 18 ml/min/1.73m^2)
Child: 109 (female) or 124 (male) ml/min/1.73 m^2
Adult males: 85–125 ml/min/1.73 m^2
Adult females: 75–115 ml/min/1.73 m^2

Glucose (S, P) (see Chapter 38)
Premature infants: 20–80 mg/dl
Full-term infants: 30–100 mg/dl
Children and adults (fasting): 60–105 mg/dl

γ-Glutamyl Transpeptidase (S)
0–1 mo: 12–27 IU/L
1–2 mo: 9–159 IU/L
2–4 mo: 7–98 IU/L
4–7 mo: 5–45 IU/L
7–15 mo: 3–30 IU/L
Adult males: 9–69 IU/L
Adult females: 3–33 IU/L

Glycohemoglobin (Hemoglobin A_{1C}) (B)
Normal: 6.3%–8.2% of total hemoglobin
Well-controlled diabetic patients ordinarily have levels < 10%

Hematocrit (B) (see Chap. 29)
At birth: 44%–64%
14–90 days: 35%–49%
6 mo–1 yr: 30%–40%
4–10 yr: 31%–43%

Immunoglobins (S)

Age	IgG	IgA (mg/dl)	IgM
2 wk–3 mo	299–852	3–66	15–149
3–6 mo	142–988	4–90	18–118
6–12 mo	418–1142	14–95	43–223
1–6 yr	356–1381	13–209	37–239
6–12 yr	625–1598	29–384	50–278
> 12 yr	660–1548	81–252	45–256

Iron (S, P)
Newborns: 20–157 μg/dl
3–9 yr: 20–141 μg/dl
9–14 yr: 21–151 μg/dl
14–16 yr: 20–181 μg/dl
Adults: 44–196 μg/dl

Iron-Binding Capacity (S, P)
Newborns: 59–175 μg/dl
Children and adults: 275–458 μg/dl

Lactate Dehydrogenase (LDH) (S, P)
Newborns (1–3 days): 40–348 IU/L
1 mo–5 yr: 150–360 IU/L
5–12 yr: 130–300 IU/L
12–16 yr: 130–280 IU/L
Adult males: 70–178 IU/L
Adult females: 42–166 IU/L

Magnesium (S, P)
Newborns: 1.5–2.3 mEq/L
Adults: 1.4–2 mEq/L

Partial Thromboplastin Time (PTT) (P)
Children: 42–54 seconds (varies with control)

Phosphorus, Inorganic (S, P)
Full-term infants:
At birth: 5–7.8 mg/dl
1–10 yr: 3.6–6.2 mg/dl
Adults: 3.1–5.1 mg/dl

Potassium (S, P)
Premature infants: 4.5–7.2 mEq/L
Full-term infants: 3.7–5.2 mEq/L
Children and adults: 3.5–5.8 mEq/L

Protein (see overleaf)

Prothrombin Time (P)
Children: 11–15 seconds (varies with control)

Sodium (S, P)
Children and adults: 135–148 mEq/L

Urea Nitrogen (BUN) (S, P)
< 2 yr: 5–15 mg/dl
> 2 yr: 10–20 mg/dl

Protein (S)

Age	Total protein	Albumin	α_1 globulin	(g/dl)	α_2 globulin	β globulin	γ globulin
Birth	4.6–7.0	3.2–4.8	0.1–0.3		0.2–0.3	0.3–0.6	0.6–1.2
3 mo	4.5–6.5	3.2–4.8	0.1–0.3		0.3–0.7	0.3–0.7	0.2–0.7
>1 yr	5.4–8.0	3.7–5.7	0.1–0.3		0.4–1.1	0.4–1.0	0.2–1.3

(Reproduced by permission from Barkin RM and Rosen P: *Emergency Pediatrics: A Guide to Ambulatory Care* (3rd ed.), St. Louis: C. V. Mosby Co., 1990)

E Frequently Used Pediatric Drugs

Antibiotics

Drug / Preparation	Dosage
Amoxicillin (Amoxil, Larotid)	
Susp: 125, 250 mg/5 ml	50 mg/kg/24 hr q 8 hr PO
Cap: 125, 250 mg	Dose: 15 mg/kg/dose tid
	Adult: 250–500 mg dose
Ampicillin (Omnipen, Polycillin)	
Susp: 125, 250 mg/5 ml	75 mg/kg/24 hr q 6 hr PO
Cap: 250, 500 mg	Dose: 20 mg/kg/dose qid
	Adult: 250–500 mg/dose
Augmentin (amoxicillin/clavulanic acid)	
Susp: 125 mg AMX/31.25 mg CLA/5 ml; 250 mg AMX/62.5 mg CLA/5 ml	30–50 mg AMX/kg/24 hr q 8 hr PO
Tab: 250, 500 mg AMX/125 mg CLA	Dose: 10–15 mg AMX/kg/dose tid
	Adult: 250–500 mg AMX/dose
	(NOTE: dosing by amoxicillin)
Cephalosporins: cephalexin (Keflex); cephradine (Velosef); cefaclor (Ceclor)	
Susp: 125, 250 mg/5 ml	40 mg/kg/24 hr q 6 hr PO
Cap: 250, 500 mg	Dose: 10 mg/kg/dose qid
	Adult: 250–500 mg/dose
Dicloxacillin (Dynapen)	
Susp: 62.5 mg/5 ml	40 mg/kg/24 hr q 6 hr PO
Cap: 125, 250 mg	Dose: 10 mg/kg/dose qid
	Adult: 250 mg/dose
Erythromycin (Pediamycin, EES, Erythrocin, E-Mycin)	
Susp: 200, 400 mg/5 ml	40 mg/kg/24 hr q 6 hr PO
Chew cap: 200 mg	Dose: 10 mg/kg/dose qid
Tab: 250, 400, 500 mg	Adult: 250–500 mg/dose
Erythromycin/sulfisoxazole (Pediazole)	
Susp: 200 mg ERY/600 mg SXZ/5 ml	40 mg ERY/120 mg SXZ/kg/24 hr q 6 hr PO
	Dose: 10 mg ERY/30 mg SXZ/kg/dose qid
Penicillin V (Pen-Vee, V-Cillin K)	
Susp: 125 mg (200,000 units), 250 mg (400,000 units)/5 ml	40 mg (65,000 units)/kg/24 hr q 6 hr PO
Tab: 125, 250 mg	Dose: 10 mg (15,000 units)/kg/dose qid
	Adult: 250–500 mg/dose

Penicillin G benzathine/penicillin G procaine (C-R Bicillin 900/300 in 2 ml)

Weight (lb)	Benzathine pen G (Bicillin LA)	Benzathine/procaine pen G (Bicillin C-R 900/300)
<30	300,000 units	300,000:100,000 units
31–60	600,000 units	600,000:200,000 units
61–90	900,000 units	900,000:300,000 units
>90	1,200,000 units	Not available

Sulfisoxazole (Gantrisin)

Susp: 500 mg/5 ml Tab: 500 mg	120 mg/kg/24 hr q 6 hr PO Dose: 30 mg/kg/dose qid Adult: 500 mg/dose

Trimethoprim-sulfamethoxazole (Bactrim, Septra)

Susp: 40 mg TMP/200 mg SMX/5 ml Tab: 80 mg TMP/400 mg SMX, 160 mg TMP/800 mg SMX	10 mg TMP/50 mg SMX/kg/24 hr q 12 hr PO Dose: 5 mg TMP/25 mg SMX/kg/dose bid Adult: 80–160 mg TMP/400–800 mg SMX/dose

Antihistamines

Diphenhydramine (Benadryl)

Susp: 12.5 mg/5 ml Cap: 25, 50 mg	5 mg/kg/24 hr q 6 hr PO Dose: 1.5 mg/kg/dose qid Adult: 25–50 mg/dose

Hydroxyzine (Atarax, Vistaril)

Syr/susp: 10, 25 mg/5 ml Tab (Atarax): 10, 25, 50 mg Cap (Vistaril): 25, 50, 100 mg	2 mg/kg/24 hr q 6 hr PO Dose: 0.5 mg/kg/dose qid Adult: 25 mg/dose

Adrenergic Agents

Albuterol (Ventolin, Proventil) Soln: 0.5%	Nebulizer: 0.01–0.03 ml/kg/dose in 2 ml saline. May repeat. Adult: 0.5 ml/dose
Terbutaline Soln: 0.1%	0.01 ml/kg/dose SQ q 20 min prn × 3 (maximum: 0.25 ml/dose); nebulizer: 0.03 ml/kg/dose (adult: 0.5 ml/dose) in 2 ml saline q 4 hr
Epinephrine (1:1,000)	0.01 ml/kg/dose SQ q 20 min prn × 3 (maximum: 0.35 ml/dose)
Racemic epinephrine 2.25% (Micronephrine)	Nebulizer: 0.25–0.50 ml in 2.5 ml saline q 2 hr prn

Theophylline

Age	Loading dose (mg/kg)	Maintenance dose (mg/kg/hr)
<12 mo	5–6	0.7
1–9 yr	5–6	0.9
10 yr and over	5–6	0.6

Steroids

Prednisone

Tab: 5, 10, 20 mg Susp: 5 mg/5 ml	1–2 mg/kg/24 hr q 12–24 hr PO Dose: 0.5–1 mg/kg/dose bid Adult: 40–80 mg/dose

Dexamethasone (Decadron) Vial: 4, 24 mg/ml Elix: 0.5 mg/5 ml Tab: 1.5, 4, 6 mg	0.25–0.5 mg/kg/dose q 6 hr IM, IV, PO
Hydrocortisone (Solu-Cortef) Vial: 100, 250, 500 mg	4–5 mg/kg/dose q 6 hr IV, IM
Methylprednisolone (Solu-Medrol) Vial: 40, 125, 500, 1,000 mg	1–2 mg/kg/dose q 6 hr IV, IM
Anticonvulsants	
Diazepam (Valium) Tab: 2, 5, 10 mg Vial: 5 mg/ml	0.2–0.3 mg/kg/dose IV (< 1 mg/min) q 2–5 min prn Adult: 5–10 mg/dose
Lorazepam (Ativan) Vial: 2, 4 mg/ml	0.05–0.15 mg/kg/dose IV slowly Adult: 2.5 mg–10 mg/dose
Phenobarbital Elix: 20 mg/ml Tab: 15, 30, 60, 90, 100 mg Vial: 65, 130 mg/ml	Load: 10–15 mg/kg/dose PO, IM, IV (< 25–50 mg/min or < 1 mg/kg/min) Adult: 100 mg/dose IV q 20 min prn × 3 Maintenance: 3–5 mg/kg/24 hr q 12–24 hr PO Adult: 200–300 mg/24 hr
Phenytoin (Dilantin) Susp: 30, 125 mg/5 ml Tab: (chew): 50 mg Cap: 30, 100 mg Amp: 50 mg/ml	Load: 10–20 mg/kg PO, IV (< 40 mg/min or < 0.5 mg/kg/min) Adult: 800–1,200 mg Maintenance: 5–10 mg/kg/24 hr q 12–24 hr PO Adult: 200–400 mg/24 hr
Carbamazepine (Tegretol) Tab: 100 (chew), 200 mg	15–30 mg/kg/24 hr q 8–12 hr PO (maximum: 1,200–1,600 mg/24 hr)
Valproic acid (Depakene) Syr: 250 mg/5 ml Cap: 250 mg	15–60 mg/kg/24 hr q 8–24 hr PO Adult: 250–750 mg/dose tid
Ethosuximide (Zarontin) Syr: 250 mg/5 ml Cap: 250 mg	20–30 mg/kg/24 hr q 24 hr PO (maximum: 1,000 mg/24 hr)
Antipyretics/Analgesics	
Aspirin (salicylate, ASA) Tab: 81 (chew), 325 mg Supp: 65, 130, 195, 325 mg	10–15 mg/kg/dose q 4–6 hr PO Adult: 10 grains (650 mg)/dose
Acetaminophen (Tylenol, Tempra) Drop: 80 mg/0.8 ml Elix: 160 mg/5 ml Tab: 80 (chew), 160 junior, 325 mg Supp: 120, 325 mg	10–15 mg/kg/dose q 4–6 hr PO Adult: 10 grains (650 mg)/dose

Codeine	
Elix: 10 mg/5 ml (with antitussive), 12 mg/5 ml (with 120 mg acetaminophen)	0.5 mg/kg/dose q 4–6 hr PO, IM Adult: 30–60 mg/dose
Tab: 15, 30, 60 mg	
Vial: 30, 60 mg	
DTP (lytic) cocktail	
Meperidine (Demerol) plus	1 mg/kg (maximum: 50 mg/dose)
promethazine (Phenergan) plus	0.25 mg/kg
chlorpromazine (Thorazine)	0.25 mg/kg (give in one syringe deep IM; may double per kg dose)
Meperidine/hydroxyzine	
Meperidine (Demerol) plus	1 mg/kg/dose
hydroxyzine (Atarax, Vistaril)	0.5 mg/kg/dose IM (give in one syringe)
Poisoning	
Ipecac, syrup	6–12 mo: 10 ml 1–12 yr: 15 ml >12 yr: 30 ml May repeat in children >12 mo if no vomiting after 20 min; give fluids
Magnesium sulfate	250 mg/kg/dose PO Adult: 20 g/dose PO
Activated charcoal	
Mix with magnesium sulfate and water (100–200 ml) and flavoring	10–30 g/dose PO Adult: 30–100 g/dose PO

(Modified from Barkin RM and Rosen P: *Emergency Pediatrics: A Guide to Ambulatory Care* (3rd ed.), St. Louis: C.V. Mosby Co., 1990.)

F Parental Instruction Guide

These parental instruction guides may provide valuable information in reviewing common approaches to problems routinely seen in children. The format should facilitate an understanding of common therapeutic intervention and may be useful for the clinician as well as the parent.

NOTE: These guides were initially developed in conjunction with the Rose Children's Center, Rose Medical Center, Denver CO. They serve as a guideline for treating medical problems. Specific management and further information must be individualized by the treating care provider.

Abdominal Pain

Sudden abdominal or belly pain often results from problems that may improve without medical attention. However, several problems can be potentially life threatening and require immediate action. (See also Chap. 20.)

What to Look for

Belly or abdominal pain can be described by its location, nature, and associated problems.

Locate the pain. Different places are associated with specific problems. Although this is often difficult to do, finding out where the pain is may narrow down the problem. For instance, the liver is in the upper right part of the abdomen, the spleen in the upper left section, the stomach more central, and the kidneys in the lower part, the latter often causing pain in the lower back.

The pain may be throughout the belly. This is common in gastroenteritis (stomach flu) with vomiting or diarrhea, as well as with abdominal muscle strain from an injury, hard coughing or constipation.

Describe the nature of the pain as steady, sharp, intermittent or crampy. Determine if the pain is getting worse, improving or remaining constant. Describe things that make the pain worse or better.

If the pain is associated with **vomiting** or **diarrhea**, determine the appearance, amount, and color of the material, as well as any presence of blood. Blood in the vomitus (red or "coffee grounds") implies that there is irritation or ulceration, while bloody stool (red or "black tarry") may result from a tear (fissure) of the rectum, allergy to soy or cow's milk, irritation of the lower bowel or damage to the intestines.

Appendicitis causes severe, sharp pain, beginning in the center of the belly and then moving to the lower right area. The belly is painful to touch, often hurting more on release after pushing in with your hand. In many children, particularly those under two years, it is difficult to make this diagnosis. A fever with vomiting, nausea and poor appetite is common.

When to Call Your Child's Doctor

CALL IMMEDIATELY IF:

Severe belly pain lasting over six hours
Severe pain with marked tenderness when the abdomen is touched, especially when the hand is released, that decreases when your child bends over or if your child is under one year of age
Moderate pain that is getting worse
Blood in vomitus or stool (digested blood looks black and tarry)
Green (bile-stained) material in vomitus
Recent injury to belly
Change in mental alertness
Rapid or shallow breathing
Very sick appearance
Possible drug or poison ingestion

CALL WITHIN A FEW HOURS, USUALLY FOLLOWING HOME TREATMENT, IF:

Pain lasts over 24 hours or localizes to one part of the abdomen
Fever over 100°F (38.3°C) that lasts for 24 hours
Signs of dehydration (loss of water) including decreased urination, less moisture in diapers, dry mouth, no tears, weight loss, sleepiness or irritability
Jaundice (yellow skin or eyes)
Painful, bloody or increased frequency of urination

CALL FOR AN APPOINTMENT IF:

Recurrent pain

What You Can Do

If your child has none of the symptoms listed under "Call immediately," watch your child carefully for several hours. During this period, treat any vomiting or diarrhea with the usual, home approaches.

Give small sips of clear liquids while allowing your child to rest
Treat fever with acetaminophen. Avoid aspirin, laxatives and other medications not recommended by your doctor. Do not give pain medicines
Evaluate your child for changes every two hours. If your child does not improve, or worsens during a 12- to 24-hour period, call your doctor

Caution

Do not delay calling if there has been a rapid onset of severe abdominal pain
Bloody (or tarry) stools require evaluation immediately; watch for dehydration (loss of water)
Watch the nature of the pain and the degree of sickness closely; contact your doctor again if either increases

Anemia

Children with blood that has a low proportion of red blood cells (hematocrit) are anemic. The most common cause in children under two years of age is iron deficiency because of an inadequate diet. Loss of blood from bleeding or abnormal breakdown of blood (hemolysis) may also cause anemia. (See also Chap. 29.)

What to Look for

Mild anemia usually has no signs or symptoms. If severe, your child may be weak, tired, irritable and pale. Older children may behave differently or have learning or developmental problems. With very severe anemia, children are short of breath and have a rapid heart rate.

When to Call Your Child's Doctor

CALL IMMEDIATELY IF:

Shortness of breath or rapid pulse

CALL WITHIN A FEW HOURS IF:

Unusual weakness, tiredness or irritability

What You Can Do

If there is an iron deficiency, change your child's diet to include more iron-rich foods such as meats, eggs, green vegetables and enriched cereals and breads. If your child is an infant, restrict milk intake to a maximum of 24 ounces per day.

Initially, iron drops (Fer-in-Sol) should be taken as prescribed. Your child's blood will be rechecked in one to two weeks and again at one and two months to be certain that the anemia is improving. The stool may become black.

Visiting Your Child's Doctor

After an initial dietary assessment, a physical examination may reveal evidence of anemia. If your doctor does not think the anemia is due to an unbalanced diet and low iron, potential sources of bleeding or blood breakdown will be explored.

A hematocrit or hemoglobin test provides a measure of the anemia. Evaluation of red blood cells should confirm an iron deficiency. If the cause is uncertain, your doctor may consult a specialist in blood cells (hematologist).

Caution

Change the diet to include iron-rich foods while giving extra iron if prescribed.

Asthma

Asthma is due to constriction and narrowing of the lower airway, often with inflammation and swelling of the airway. Allergies as well as infection or irritants in the air, such as dust or chemicals, may cause this. Wheezing often follows a respiratory infection or cold.

What to Look for

Asthmatic children breathe with a rapid rate and wheezing (high-pitched sound in the chest, not rattling in the back of the throat). There may also be congestion, cough or fever. Some children may have only a prolonged cough.

In more serious cases, your child may develop difficult and rapid breathing, exaggerated movement of the chest and blueness of the lips and fingers (cyanosis). With worsening, your child may have difficulty speaking or may become restless or sleepy. Complications may include lung infections with the sputum changing from white to yellow or green, or dehydration (loss of water) due to poor fluid intake.

Wheezing may be due to other problems such as pneumonia or the inhaling of fluid and foreign material into the lungs.

When to Call Your Child's Doctor

CALL IMMEDIATELY IF:

Breathing becomes more difficult or is not improving
Blue or dusky lips or nails
Difficulty speaking because of shortness of breath
Restlessness or excessive sleepiness

CALL WITHIN A FEW HOURS IF:

Breathing is getting worse, but there is no real distress
Signs of dehydration (loss of water) including decreased urination, less moisture in diapers, dry mouth, no tears, weight loss, sleepiness or irritability
Recent hospitalization for asthma
Steroids such as prednisone taken in the last year
Not improving after 24 hours of therapy
Persistent fever for the last 24 hours
Difficulty sleeping
Change of sputum from white to yellow or green
Medications not tolerated

CALL FOR AN APPOINTMENT IF:

There is a persistent cough
No resolution after two days

What You Can Do

Keep your child calm by rocking, holding and being reassuring. Reduce activity and encourage warm fluids. Fluids are essential and often accepted in small sips; don't worry if your child doesn't take solids for a day or so. Keep track of whether your child is improving or getting worse. Make sure medications are taken, if prescribed.

You may have to give your child asthma medicines, commonly prescribed to be given every six hours (first dose is usually 1-½ times the regular dose) unless slow-release preparation is used. If the problem is caused by an infection or specific exposure, such as dust, continue the medicine for at least 72 hours after the wheezing has ceased. If the problem is recurrent, your child may need prolonged medication, often using sustained-release forms, which require less frequent administration. The asthma medicines may cause vomiting or irritability, requiring a dosage change.

A special inhalation machine or pocket, hand-held inhaler may be used three to four times per day. This may be done in conjunction with other asthma medicines.

Ongoing therapy often requires a combination of asthma medicines, nebulizers (inhalation machines for medicine), avoidance of substances that trigger the attack, and occasionally, desensitization shots by an allergist. Be certain to remove bothersome asthma items from the home.

If any adults in the household smoke, discuss the importance of not exposing your child to "passive smoking." Stop smoking.

Caution

Do not give more medication than prescribed. Asthma medications can cause side effects.

Bites – Animal and Human

What to Look for

The bite will produce puncture wounds or damage to the skin or underlying tissue. Things to consider in deciding if a bite is serious include:

1. **Location and depth of the wound.**
   See if there is an injury to the deeper tissues or just a scrape. Bites to the hands, feet or face are serious, even if the wound looks minor.
2. **Animal bites.**
   Rabies may result from bites of skunks, foxes, coyotes, raccoons, wild dogs and cats, and bats. If a domestic dog or cat is sick or the attack was unprovoked, rabies should be considered. Rodents such as mice, rats, squirrels, hamsters, gophers, chipmunks, rabbits and hares do not normally carry rabies. If there is any question, the public health department can provide information about the local animal population.
3. **Human bites.**
   However innocuous or rare, children should be watched closely for infection.
4. **Infection.**
   Animal and human bites may become red, swollen, acutely tender or pus-filled. Children may develop a fever or become seriously ill and require immediate attention. When infection does occur, it usually does so within three days of the bite.
   Children must have a current tetanus immunization (five years for a major injury and 10 years for a minor wound).

When to Call Your Child's Doctor

CALL IMMEDIATELY IF:

Biting animal can carry rabies (see above)
Animal is sick or the bite was unprovoked
Bite is on the face, hands or feet
Bite produces a great deal of damage or bleeding, or bite is deep

CALL WITHIN A FEW HOURS IF:

Wound may require sutures
Wound looks red, tender, swollen, drains pus or your child develops a fever
Tetanus immunization has lapsed
Prescribed medications are not tolerated

What You Can Do

Thorough cleansing is probably the most important part of treatment. If there is bleeding, apply direct pressure on the wound; if not, wash the injury with soap and water for at least five minutes. Watch the bite closely for infection over the next three to five days

Update tetanus status

If the rabies status of the animal is unknown and rabies is a consideration, try to capture the animal and have the public health department observe it in isolation for 10 days

Most importantly, instruct your children not to play with unfamiliar animals or place their faces near dogs

Teach your children to play calmly and avoid frightening animals with loud sounds or unexpected, quick movements

Do not leave children unattended with dogs and other potentially dangerous animals

Caution

Careful examination of the region of animal or human bites is necessary to determine if there is damage to deep tissues; look for infection

Bloody Nose

The blood vessels in the nose can bleed due to minimal injury or irritation, particularly in dry climates. A bloody nose is common after minimal injury from a cold or from nose picking. (See also Chap. 16.)

What to Look for

This occurs more commonly in winter in areas of low humidity. Occasionally, bleeding can occur from a foreign body in the nose, usually accompanied by an odor and drainage from the nostril. A bleeding problem can cause nosebleeds, but bleeding and bruising also occur elsewhere.

When to Call Your Child's Doctor

CALL WITHIN A FEW HOURS IF:

Continuing bleeding after constant and uninterrupted pressure for a minimum of two 10-minute periods for a total of 20 minutes.

CALL FOR AN APPOINTMENT IF:

Recurrent nosebleeds
Accompanying bruises

What You Can Do

Have your child blow his/her nose to remove clots. Then compress the soft and bony part of the nose downward toward the cheeks with thumb and forefinger for a minimum of 10 minutes. If this fails, hold the nose for an additional 10 minutes. Do not interrupt these periods to inspect the area. Keep your child calm by holding him/her on your lap, stroking the forehead and being reassuring. Optimally, have your child in a sitting position to minimize swallowing blood.

Reduce the frequency of future nosebleeds by placing petrolatum (Vaseline) or other ointment just inside the nostrils daily for four to five days. Use a cold-air vaporizer at night.

Visiting Your Child's Doctor

Your doctor will have your child sit or lie down with his/her head back (depending on age and level of cooperation) and will perform compression of the nose, even if this has been done at home. Rarely is gauze packing or electric cautery necessary.

Burns

Childhood burns can result from electrical contact, hot objects, hot water and other liquids, fires, chemicals and sunburn.

What to Look for

Factors to consider in children with burns include the amount of skin burned, depth and location of the burn and how the burn occurred.

1. **Amount of skin burned.**
   The larger the area or body surface of the burn, the more severe. Your doctor should see your child if there are burns over 5 percent of the body. Children with burns over more than 10 percent of their body often require hospitalization.
   Approximations may be inexact. In general, particularly in older children and adults, each arm is about 9 percent of the body surface, each leg 18 percent, the chest and back 18 percent each, and the head and neck 9 percent.
2. **Depth of the burn.**
   First-degree burns have only reddening of the skin such as in sunburns;
   Second-degree burns result in redness and fluid under the skin, forming blisters. They usually heal well but can produce complications such as fluid loss and infection;
   Third-degree burns produce injury to the deep layers of the skin. The skin has a hard, brownish surface, appearing charred. Often there is no feeling. These burns cause scarring and need specialized grafting.
3. **Location.**
   Burns involving the hands, face, eyes, ears, feet or genital area are particularly difficult to care for without specialized help.
4. **Mechanism.**
   How the burn occurred can influence the type of injury to be expected.

When to Call Your Child's Doctor

CALL IMMEDIATELY IF:

Second-degree burns cover more than 5 percent of the body surface
Any third-degree burns are present
Burns of the hands, face, eyes, ears, feet or genital area
Burns result from a fire in a closed space
Shortness of breath or rapid breathing
Burns result from an electrical source
Burns are caused from either acids or caustics
Explanation of how the burn occurred is suspicious (exclude child abuse)
Other medical problems exist

CALL WITHIN A FEW HOURS IF:

Second-degree burns cover less than 5 percent of the body surface
First-degree burns cover more than 5 percent of the body surface
Increasingly painful burns, with tenderness, redness or draining pus develops
Tetanus immunization status is uncertain or needs updating

What You Can Do

Remove clothing and apply cool water over the burn area using clean towels or cloths to reduce the amount of skin damage and pain. If the burn is totally first-degree, red and tender only, involves less than 10 percent of the surface area, this initial treatment is probably adequate.

Second-degree burns require more care. Blisters should be left intact. Remove the loose skin from broken blisters using clean tweezers – your doctor should handle this for large-area burns.

If the burn is a very small (1 to 4 percent) second-degree burn and does not require a doctor's visit, use an antibiotic ointment or cream or leave the wound open to the air. If prescribed by your doctor, use a special burn cream, Silvadene, and cover with a nonsticky dressing. Redress the burn in 24 hours and then every two to three days for a period of 10 to 14 days. If the bandage sticks, soak it in warm water before removing. While redressing, cleanse the surface with soap and water. Keep the dressing clean and dry. Elevate the extremity immediately to limit swelling and protect the area from further injury. Continue elevation for 24 to 48 hours or until you visit your child's doctor.

Treat tar burns by removing the tar with mineral oil and then treating as any other burn.

Electrical burns require evaluation by a doctor to determine the nature of the injury. Remove your child from the source, being careful to avoid electrical shock. If your child bites an electrical cord with a subsequent burn to the lip, your doctor should evaluate and watch the area closely.

Chemical burns initially require copious washing at the scene, usually before transport. Wash off or remove all contaminated clothing and rinse your child using a shower, hose or tub. Rinse eyes first if involved.

Prevention is the key to minimizing the frequency of burns.

Protect fireplaces, heating devices and hot objects, hide matches, discard flammable liquids, turn down water heaters to 120 degrees, and be alert to potential accidents. Install early smoke detection devices and fire extinguishers in high-risk areas. Develop an escape plan and conduct drills.

Caution

Second-degree burns over 5 percent of the body surface require evaluation, particularly if they include areas that are difficult to treat. Evidence of respiratory distress requires evaluation. Electrical and chemical burns require specific intervention.

Cold or Upper Respiratory Infection (URI)

Colds are common in children, increasing in number as your children come in contact with others, particularly in day-care settings. Preschoolers can have up to five to eight colds per year. Viruses cause colds.

What to Look for

Your child may have congestion with a runny or stuffy nose, often with a sore throat, posterior nasal drip, cough, headache, red eyes, hoarseness or fever. He/she may have a poor appetite and be sleepy and irritable. Muscles are often tender and may ache. Occasionally, colds lead to complications such as ear infections or pneumonia.

When to Call Your Child's Doctor

CALL IMMEDIATELY IF:

Difficult or rapid breathing
Marked irritability or listlessness

CALL WITHIN A FEW HOURS IF:

Ear pain
Chest pain
Sore throat with or without white spots on tonsils
No improvement or persistent fever after 72 hours
Infant is under three months of age
Skin under the nose becomes raw or cracked, often with golden crusting
Discharge from the nose becomes green and contains pus

What You Can Do

Colds require little therapy. To make your child more comfortable, take the following steps. In the younger child, use water nosedrops to reduce congestion, then clean the nose with a bulb syringe (usually given to parents when their child is born). In the older child, decongestants and antihistamines, such as Actifed, Rondec or Dimetapp may offer relief, particularly if the problem is a runny nose. A cold-air vaporizer may reduce the symptoms.

Fever medicine such as acetaminophen (Tylenol, Tempra, etc.) should be used to keep the temperature relatively normal. Antibiotics are not needed.

Encourage and push fluids. It is not crucial that your child eat any solids for a day or two until the cold resolves somewhat; fluids are essential! Clear fluids are often tolerated well. Specific products that are ideal for infants include Lytren and Pedialyte. Products available at home include Gatorade, soda (defizzed at room temperature) and liquid Jell-O (one package mixed with a quart instead of a pint of water).

Colic

Prolonged periods of fussiness occurring repeatedly over several days are noted in up to 10 percent of children, usually between two weeks and three months of life. This is normal. Little is known about this condition, but it is thought to be caused by gas-like abdominal pains. Many people think it occurs in children who are particularly sensitive to stimuli. It is a benign condition that resolves spontaneously when babies get older. (See also Chap. 9.)

What to Look for

Children cry and are irritable at a similar time of each day, the evening being most common. Babies are difficult to console and may draw their legs up. A number of steps are useful but may not always calm the child. In between episodes, babies are consolable.

Other causes of irritability can include dirty diapers, hunger, illness, diaper pin(s) sticking the child, teething, drug poisoning and unrecognized injuries or illness.

When to Call Your Child's Doctor

CALL WITHIN A FEW HOURS IF:

Vomiting or diarrhea
Crying that lasts over four hours
Fever, runny nose, cough or vomiting
Baby is younger than two weeks or older than four months
Parents are tired and getting increasingly frustrated

What You Can Do

First, make sure that there is no specific cause for crying (e.g., pin in clothing or thread around a toe). Then, use any number of activities to console the baby. Rhythmic activities such as rocking, automatic swings, rides or walking are often helpful. Try cuddling your child, wrapping him/her in a Snugli, playing soothing music or giving him/her a pacifier for sucking. Each child responds uniquely. It is important to discover those things that are useful for your particular infant.

On occasion, you must allow your child to just cry him/herself to sleep. Make sure that your child is not hungry (i.e., has eaten in the last 2 to 2½ hours), that the nipple was not plugged and that the diaper is not dirty. You may have difficulty listening to your child crying, but responding every time gets tiresome very quickly and encourages your child to be increasingly demanding. All children prefer being held, rocked or fed constantly, and crying is often an attempt to get this. Setting some limits and making the decision not to respond every time your baby cries will discourage increasingly demanding behavior. This is important for parents and for children! Reach a reasonable balance and discuss it with your doctor. Talk with others about your frustrations. Remember who is supposed to be in control!

Constipation

Children have many patterns of bowel movements. They *normally* have infrequent movements, sometimes going once every three to four days. Children may develop problems when there is pain or discomfort with bowel movements. Dietary changes can cause constipation. A change in bowel pattern, rather than the number of days between movements, is of greatest importance. (See also Chap. 22.)

What to Look for

Pain or discomfort with bowel movements can occur with hard stools or, more frequently, when there is a tear (fissure) in the rectum. The stool may have bright-red blood streaks. Rarely, patients with severe diaper rash will withhold bowel movements due to pain.

Beyond the infant period, constipation may occur when toilet training begins and parents are giving a great deal of attention to bowel movements. Your child may retain stool, often for so long that he/she develops crampy abdominal (belly) pain, usually increasing temporarily after stooling.

In older children, stool retention may recur due to emotional factors and stress. These children often have abdominal pain, again decreasing partially with movements.

If retention occurs over a long enough period, liquid stools may develop around the hardened mass and leak out.

When to Call Your Child's Doctor

CALL WITHIN A FEW HOURS IF:

Painful bowel movements
Blood in stool
No stool for five days
Abdominal pain for more than two hours

CALL FOR AN APPOINTMENT, USUALLY AFTER BEGINNING HOME TREATMENT, IF:

Recurrent abdominal pain
Soiling
Tear or fissure around rectum
Medications contributing to problem
Associated with toilet training

What You Can Do

Changing the diet is usually sufficient. For your baby, give one tablespoon of Karo syrup (light or dark) in every four to eight ounces of formula, milk or water. Encourage foods like prune juice and strained apricots, peaches, pears, prunes and other fruits when appropriate.

Be supportive, particularly if the problem is related to toilet training. Slow down and let your child do it at his/her own pace.

Encourage older children to drink prune juice and to eat bran products. Push fruits and vegetables and other sources of fiber and roughage such as celery, oranges, bran flakes, prunes, figs, dates, peaches, and pears. Fluid intake is essential. Discourage milk products, bananas and applesauce, since they are constipating.

On rare occasions, use natural laxatives, such as Maltsupex or Metamucil, usually starting with a dose of one-half to one tablespoon twice a day and increasing as necessary.

Treat rectal tears by softening the stool and keeping the area dry. Apply a cream after diaper changes to soothe.

Do not use enemas and suppositories; they can be dangerous.

Convulsions or Seizures

A seizure (convulsion) is a transient disturbance of brain function, usually caused by an area of irritation in the brain. There are many forms of convulsions and many causes. For children who have had convulsions in the past, the most common cause for a recurrence is forgetting to take a few doses of anti-seizure medicines.

The vast majority of seizures are known as *febrile seizures* and occur in 2–5 percent of *normal* children as a result of a high fever. They usually stop by themselves and do not cause any long-term problems.

(See also Chap. 36.)

What to Look for

Convulsions commonly cause a jerking movement of the extremities, with associated rolling of the eyes, and loss of control of urine and stool. One side of the body may be more affected than the other. Children are not usually responsive or aware of what is going on during the convulsion. Breathing difficulty may occur. Although most convulsions are self-limited and last only 60 to 90 seconds, episodes may go on for some time until medicines are given and the seizures are stopped. Following a convulsion, children are usually sleepy and rest for a period.

Recall if your child has had a fever or been sick, has experienced recent head injury, or has possibly taken any drugs. Ascertain if there is a history of past convulsions either in the child or in members of the immediate family. If anti-seizure medications are normally taken, it is important to determine if all doses have been taken.

A child having a *febrile seizure* usually also has a fever, most commonly caused by a cold or ear infection. The convulsions usually involve all extremities, and stop without therapy within 15 minutes. The seizure is often the first time you realize that your child is sick.

Rarely, children with seizures have episodes of staring or unusual movement of the face, tongue or mouth.

When to Call Your Child's Doctor

CALL IMMEDIATELY (CALL 911) IF:

Child's first seizure
Convulsion still going on
Difficulty breathing
Blue color of skin, lips, fingernails
Child has fever
Child not awake and alert

CALL WITHIN A FEW HOURS IF:

Any seizure, if stopped spontaneously
Child having trouble taking anti-seizure medications
Episode of staring or unusual movement of the face, tongue or mouth
Child has febrile seizure, was evaluated and now has a prolonged temperature (for more than 36 hours) or is exhibiting behavioral changes, vomiting, headache, stiff neck or nonblanching rash

What You Can Do

First, make sure that your child can breathe as easily as possible by putting his/her head in the "sniff" position to open the airway as much as possible. If your child is having great trouble breathing or has stopped breathing, start using rescue breathing techniques.

Try to make sure that your child doesn't hurt him/herself by striking his/her arm, leg or head. If your child's mouth is open, insert something soft like a washcloth to prevent the teeth from clenching tightly.

Arrange for rapid transport of your child to the hospital for treatment of the convulsions and evaluation of their cause, unless there is a history of recurrences.

If your child has a fever and is slowly waking up from the convulsion, begin medicines to bring the fever down.

When mildly ill or running a low grade fever, the child with febrile seizures should receive acetaminophen in appropriate doses early in the course. The ill child should avoid dangerous situations including bathing in a bathtub unattended, swimming, climbing on a jungle gym, swinging, bicycle riding, operating machinery, using sharp utensils, etc.

Visiting Your Child's Doctor

The first priority is to give oxygen to make sure that your child is breathing normally. Your doctor will then attempt to stop the seizures, if they are ongoing, by using any one of a number of medications.

Attention will then turn to prevention of recurrences and assessment to determine the cause of the seizures. This will involve a number of blood, X-ray and other tests, depending on the various causes that are being considered.

If your child had a febrile seizure, your doctor will review with you that this type is usually harmless and occurs in 2 to 5 percent of normal children. There is only a very slight increased risk of developing seizures later on. Rarely are there any long-term problems. Anti-seizure medications are rarely used. The visit to your doctor will focus on bringing down your child's temperature using Tylenol, Tempra, etc., and determining what infection your child has that caused the high fever. Common infections, as well as serious infections of the nervous system, will be considered.

Caution

Make sure your child's airway is open and breathing is adequate. Your doctor should see your child to determine the cause of the seizure, even if it has stopped.

Cough

An irritation of the airway or lungs causes coughing, which serves as a protective reflex to prevent mucus or pus from accumulating. Coughing is only a symptom; it is important to define the cause. (See also Chap. 44.)

What to Look for

A runny nose, sore throat and fever often accompany a cough. Allergy or irritation of the posterior throat may cause a dry, hacking, tickling cough. A posterior nasal drip tends to cause coughs that are worse at night when your child is lying down.

Coughing is sometimes a sign of lung problems. If accompanied by rapid breathing, coughing can mean there is pneumonia, particularly if your child has a fever. Children with asthma may have a cough, and it may be the only symptom that parents notice.

Young children may inhale small objects such as toys, peanuts and raisins without being noticed by parents. This can produce immediate problems or may result in only a chronic cough and some minimal wheezing.

Croup has a unique cough that sounds like a "barking seal." Your child may have stridor (a harsh sound when he/she breathes), exaggerated chest movement and distress.

When to Call Your Child's Doctor

CALL IMMEDIATELY IF:

Shortness of breath, rapid breathing rate or difficulty breathing
Blueness of lips or nails
Breathing stopped, even momentarily
Spasms that cause choking, passing out, a bluish color of lips or persistent vomiting
Blood in sputum or mucus
Sudden onset of violent coughing in a child who might have inhaled a small object. Any other suggestion of foreign body inhalation

CALL WITHIN A FEW HOURS IF:

Wheezing
Croupy, "barking seal" type cough with any difficulty breathing
Minimal increase in breathing rate
Fever for more than 72 hours
Your child is younger than three months
Produces yellowish-green material
Chest pain
Vomiting occurs repeatedly with coughing

CALL FOR AN APPOINTMENT IF:

Lasts more than two weeks
Interferes with sleep

What You Can Do

Treatment depends on the type and cause of the cough. Children over four years can suck on cough drops or hard candy. You can make a good soothing mixture at home by mixing equal amounts of honey (corn syrup for children under one year) and lemon concentrate. Also use warm liquids such as tea.

Cough syrups are rarely useful, although some expectorants may loosen secretions. Very rarely, when the cough is interfering with sleep, work or school, or causing vomiting or chest pain, your doctor may prescribe a stronger cough medicine containing dextromethorphan (DM) or codeine. Use these with caution because they reduce the protection that coughing gives the lungs. They will not eliminate coughing entirely.

Coughs due to posterior nasal drip worsen at night. Give decongestants before bedtime; use a cold-air vaporizer in your child's bedroom. Encourage fluid intake. Minimize or eliminate smoking from the house.

Croup

Inflammation of the airway at the voice box causes difficulty breathing. It is usually due to a virus.

What to Look for

Children with croup are usually under three years and develop a cough that sounds like a "barking seal" preceded by a runny nose, cough, hoarseness and fever. Croup generally gets worse in the middle of the night between 2:00 and 6:00 a.m. with a crowing sound while breathing. Most children emit this crowing sound only when upset or anxious. The difficulty may quickly worsen to the extent that the child is gasping for air, with marked accentuation of chest movement. Croup usually resolves over a period of three to four days.

More worrisome is the child who rapidly develops a crowing sound when breathing in and out while at rest. This child may appear very sick, with a high fever, difficulty handling secretions, drooling and a preference for sitting up. These symptoms are due to inflammation of the epiglottis, which sits above the windpipe and can block air passage. In contrast to croup, epiglottis is due to a specific bacteria known as *H. influenzae* and may progress very rapidly. Rarely, children inhaling a foreign body may have a similar reaction.

When to Call Your Child's Doctor

CALL IMMEDIATELY IF:

Crowing constantly at rest or when upset
Shortness of breath, difficulty breathing or rapid respiratory rate
Increasing agitation or sleepiness
Blueness of lips or nails
Difficulty handling secretions or drooling
High fever in toxic child
Preference for sitting up with the chin protruding forward
Potential inhalation of foreign body

CALL WITHIN A FEW HOURS IF:

Crowing when child is very upset and crying
Evidence of dehydration noted by decreased amount of urination, fewer wet diapers, listlessness, irritability, or dry mucous membranes

What You Can Do

Give mist continuously. Use a vaporizer (cold preferred to reduce the risk of burns) in your child's bedroom. Use two, if needed, to generate enough mist. While this is being set up or if your child gets worse, take your child to the bathroom, close the door, run hot water to generate steam and sit or stand, soothing your child, as the steam fills the room. Do not put the child in the scalding water. If there is increasing discomfort, take your child outside; cold air may reduce the distress.

Keep your child calm by holding, rocking, reading and being soothing, while pushing fluids, often in small sips. Do not worry if your child will not take solids for a day or so; drinking is more important.

It is imperative to watch your child closely, paying particular attention to worsening breathing. This is one of the few circumstances when sleeping in your child's room may be reassuring.

Visiting Your Child's Doctor

Your doctor will evaluate the amount of breathing difficulty by determining the presence of crowing while resting or crying, the rate of breathing and the amount of accentuation of breathing movements. If there are problems at rest, your doctor will usually hospitalize your child. Your doctor may give two medications, one administered by a breathing treatment and steroids given as a shot or liquid.

Caution

When a crowing sound is present at rest, your doctor should evaluate your child. Hospitalization is usually necessary.

Diarrhea

Frequent liquid or soft stools may be normal or may represent a change due to irritation or infection of the intestines. Allergy or too many antibiotics (especially amoxicillin or ampicillin) may also contribute.

Breast-feeding often causes yellow, mushy stools up to 12 times per day after feedings; a sudden change in pattern may indicate an abnormality.

(See also Chap. 23.)

What to Look for

Infants with diarrhea have liquid, runny stools, often with enough water loss to produce a water ring around the solid material. Older children with diarrhea commonly have several runny stools per day.

Viral gastroenteritis (stomach flu) is common with children and is accompanied by fever, runny nose, and sore throat. Vomiting is frequent. Diarrhea caused by other factors can make children very sick, with marked abdominal belly cramping and pain, fatigue, and nausea. Illness can follow eating contaminated food.

The stool may contain mucus or blood.

In children with a great deal of water loss due to vomiting or diarrhea, dehydration (loss of water) may develop, particularly in those who are reluctant to take fluids.

When to Call Your Child's Doctor

CALL IMMEDIATELY IF:

Blood in stool
Severe belly cramps or vomiting for more than two hours
Increasing frequency of stools or water loss
Evidence of dehydration (loss of water) including decreased urination, less moisture in diapers, dry mouth, no tears, rapid breathing, weight loss, sleepiness, or irritability
High fever or sick and toxic looking
Vomiting clear liquids

CALL WITHIN A FEW HOURS IF:

Diarrhea increases in frequency or amount with more than 10 episodes of vomiting or diarrhea in 24 hours
Diarrhea not improving after 24 hours of taking clear liquids, or not completely gone after three to four days
Mucus in stool
Fever for more than two days (call immediately if your child is less than three months old and has a fever)
Child is taking medication

CALL FOR AN APPOINTMENT IF:

Mild diarrhea has occurred for one week or more

What You Can Do

Reduce or eliminate all solids from the diet; offer clear fluids. Children can easily go several days without solids.

Push, encourage and force liquids to make sure that too much water is not lost. Do this in a kind and supportive manner in very small amounts, particularly if there has been any vomiting. In the young child with vomiting and diarrhea, many people actually give 1 teaspoon of liquid at a time until the vomiting has at least partially resolved.

Specific products that are ideal for infants include Lytren and Pedialyte. Products available at home include Gatorade, soda (defizzed at room temperature) and liquid

Jell-O (one package mixed with a quart of water instead of a pint). If the diarrhea is mild, it is often adequate to make your child's formula half-strength by adding twice as much water; in the breastfed child, give a little supplemental water.

After a prolonged course of diarrhea, younger children should avoid milk products for one to two weeks; soy formulas (Isomil, ProSoBee, or Soyalac) are good substitutes. If on milk, merely reduce the intake of such products while substituting other fluids. Do not use boiled skim milk. Kool-Aid and similar products are not good for diarrhea because they contain few salts.

In older children, push clear liquids. Defizzed, room temperature soda is acceptable, and your child may accept it enthusiastically.

When you see some improvement on this liquid diet, induce other foods slowly. Reintroduce infants over six months to applesauce, strained bananas and carrots. Give crackers and dry toast to older children. As tolerated, start other items in your child's normal diet over the next three to four days, avoiding bran and raw fruits and vegetables.

Stop medications causing diarrhea (ampicillin or amoxicillin); call your doctor for alternatives. Drugs such as Kaopectate have no value, and, in fact, drugs such as Lomotil can cause real problems in children. Antibiotics are rarely useful.

Visiting Your Child's Doctor

Your doctor will first make sure that your child is not dehydrated. If there is evidence of problems, your doctor will want to push fluids by mouth or intravenously; hospitalization may be required. A careful history often points to likely causes of the problem.

An examination of the stool may determine the cause of the diarrhea while an analysis of the urine assesses hydration. Additional studies may be necessary if the diarrhea is an ongoing source of concern. The plan for therapy will require careful review.

Caution

Do not use boiled skim milk. Do not use anti-diarrheal medications. Push clear liquids while watching for evidence of dehydration.

Ear Pain or Infection

Ear pain is common in children and is usually caused by infection of the ear canal or the middle ear, with accumulation of fluid under pressure. Congestion blocks the normal drainage of the middle ear through the eustachian tube, allowing fluid to build up. (See also Chap. 14.)

What to Look for

Your child may have ear pain on one or both sides. Runny nose, sore throat, fever, irritability and increased crying are often present. Changing behavior or irritability are responses to pain. Ear pain may be only one part of a more serious infection. If ear infections continue untreated, the eardrum may drain pus. Rarely, children with recurrent problems will develop a hearing loss.

When there is a rapid change in altitude such as descending in an airplane or driving down a mountain, ear pain may develop. This usually gets better with swallowing or holding the nose closed while blowing.

Pain in the ear when moved or touched does not always mean the middle ear is infected. Infection or irritation of the ear canal can occur from swimmer's ear or from drainage of the middle ear through a hole in the eardrum.

When to Call Your Child's Doctor

CALL IMMEDIATELY IF:

Your child exhibits marked irritability, sleepiness, stiff neck or looks sicker than expected
High temperature over 103°F (39.9°C)
Severe pain, causing child to scream

CALL WITHIN A FEW HOURS IF:

Temperature over 101°F (38.3°C) for 12 hours
Ear pain for over one hour or tugging, rubbing or pulling ear
Drainage from ear
Pain with movement or when touching ear
After starting treatment, no improvement after 36 hours or fever present after 72 hours

CALL FOR AN APPOINTMENT IF:

There is any question of decreased hearing

What You Can Do

You can do several things to make your child more comfortable, particularly if the pain develops in the middle of the night or your doctor can't see your child for several hours. Even when your doctor starts medication, it will not work immediately. Give fever and pain medicines such as acetaminophen (Tylenol, Tempra, etc.). Apply a warm cloth over the ear to soothe your child. If there is no drainage, use ear drops to temporarily reduce the pain.

If ear pain is due to a change in altitude, swallowing, chewing gum or blowing the nose while holding it closed may provide relief. For younger children, use a teething biscuit, pacifier or bottle.

After your doctor's visit, be sure to give all prescribed medicines and return for a recheck when scheduled. Medicines often need to be refrigerated.

Although there are multiple factors that produce ear pain, one way to help prevent infection is to prevent your child from drinking from a bottle while lying down.

Eye Redness, Discharge or Pain

An infection known as "pink eye" or conjunctivitis commonly causes redness, often with discharge. Eye irritation can also cause the same symptoms. Pain may indicate the presence of a foreign body or trauma to the eye. (See also Chap. 19.)

What to Look for

Commonly, there is a pus-like discharge preceding or accompanying other respiratory symptoms such as runny nose, sore throat or low-grade fever. Often, the eye feels itchy and irritated. The discharge is sometimes thick and plentiful, causing the eye to crust over or become matted after sleeping. A thin discharge or none at all may occur if the problem is due to a virus, an allergy, an irritant in the air or a substance that comes in contact with the eye (chlorine in pool, make-up, etc.).

The eyelids are often slightly puffy and red. On occasion the eyelids and surrounding skin become red, swollen, firm and tender, indicating a skin infection.

Foreign bodies in the eye, such as small pieces of metal, dust or gravel cause a sharp, excruciating, localized pain. You can often see the material. A scratch of the cornea from something quickly touching the eye, such as a tree branch, causes a similar sensation.

When to Call Your Child's Doctor

CALL IMMEDIATELY IF:

Lid or surrounding skin red and swollen
Eye pain
Impaired, blurred or double vision
Foreign body not easily removed
Injury to the eye, potential penetration or damage from a high-speed object
Chemical splashed in the eye
Eyeball cloudy, bloody or containing sores
Discharge from eye contains pus
Child is under one month old

CALL WITHIN A FEW HOURS IF:

Clear discharge or eye redness lasting over one week
Eyes do not improve after three days of medicine

What You Can Do

Your doctor will usually prescribe some eye medicine. While your child is awake, clean the eye and use drops every two hours. To clean, gently remove the crusting with a warm, wet cotton ball. To administer drops, pull the lower lid down and place the drops in the lower lid gently. When the eye starts to improve, you can decrease the frequency to four times daily. For younger children, you may receive ointment instead of drops, which you use four times daily. Expect blurry vision with ointment. For bad or unresponsive infections, use the ointment at bedtime in conjunction with the drops.

Your child can infect other people. Use separate towels and washcloths and always wash hands carefully.

If an allergy or irritant caused your child's infection, try to avoid these substances. Often antihistamines, such as Benadryl (or equivalent), are helpful. If a chemical splashed in your child's eye, immediately wash the eye out very well and then call for advice.

If you think there may be a foreign object in the eye, pull down the lower lid and look, lifting the material off with a soft tissue. If it is still present, turn the upper eyelid back using a cotton swab and remove object, or pull the upper lid over the lower lid to remove the particle. Another approach is to rinse the eye with running water. If there is pain, your doctor should examine the eye.

Fever

An elevated temperature is above 100.4°F (38.0°C) rectally, 99.7°F (37.6°C) orally or 99°F (37.2°C) axillary. Although infection is the most frequent cause, other factors may raise the temperature including food, excess clothing, anxiety, vigorous exercise or exposure to hot environments. When in doubt, take the temperature again in an hour.

Teething does not cause marked elevations in temperature. Immunizations, such as the DTP vaccine, can cause a transient fever during 24 to 48 hours following the injection. (See also Chap. 5.)

What to Look for

Fever is only one symptom of an infection; the important thing is to find out what is causing the temperature. Your child may also have ear pain, a sore throat, a runny nose, a cough, skin changes, vomiting and diarrhea.

Children with a high fever are often irritable or tired, with a flushed face and increased heart and breathing rates. Some children with very high temperature hallucinate. These symptoms should improve when the temperature decreases; if they do not, your doctor should see your child.

Approximately 2 to 5 percent of normal children will have a convulsion with an elevated temperature. Convulsions usually occur with high temperatures and are indeed frightening; however, children usually recover from these episodes rapidly and without problems.

When to Call Your Child's Doctor

CALL IMMEDIATELY IF:

Child is under three months old
Marked change in behavior with hallucinations, irritability, listlessness, sleepiness or crying without relief
Fever over 105°F (40.5°C) rectally
Looks sicker than expected, particularly after temperature decreases
Stiff neck, bad headache or convulsion (seizure)
Fullness of soft spot in infant
Purple spots on skin
Difficulty breathing
Abdominal or belly pain
Dehydration (loss of water) with decreased urination, less moisture in diapers, dry mouth, no tears, weight loss, sleepiness or irritability

CALL WITHIN A FEW HOURS IF:

Fever over 103°F (39.5°C) in child under two years
Fever lasts longer than 48 hours
Burning on urination
Vomiting or diarrhea lasts longer than 12 hours

What You Can Do

Taking your child's temperature is important. Take *rectal* temperatures as follows:

1. Shake the thermometer down below 96.8°F (36°C);
2. Lubricate with Vaseline, cold cream or cold water;
3. Gently insert the thermometer one-half inch into rectum. Hold your child still with his/her stomach down on your lap;
4. Leave in three minutes or until silver line stops rising;
5. Read the thermometer by turning the pointed edge of the triangle slightly in each direction until you identify the top of the mercury (silver) column;

6. On the Fahrenheit thermometer each line is 0.2°F, while on the centigrade (Celsius) thermometer each line is 0.1°C.

Take an *oral* temperature in the older child (generally at least five years old), by leaving the thermometer under the tongue for three minutes, provided that your child has had nothing to drink in the last 15 minutes. *Axillary* temperatures require that the thermometer be held under a dry armpit for four to six minutes. The elbow should be held against the chest.

Digital or electronic thermometers can simplify and shorten these procedures.

FEVER MEDICINES

Rectal temperatures below 101.5°F (38.6°C) do not need to be treated unless your child is very uncomfortable or a fever is present at bedtime. If your child is acting normally, fever medicines may be delayed until the temperature is 102.2°F (39.0°C).

Acetaminophen (Tylenol, Tempra, etc.) is usually recommended every four to six hours by mouth. If your child's temperature is above 103°F (39.5°C) and does not come down quickly with acetaminophen, you may want to try sponging. Sponge your undressed child in lukewarm water (96 to 100°F). Many people prefer laying the undressed child on a towel. Another towel or washcloth soaked in lukewarm water is placed on the child and changed every one to two minutes. This is done for 15 to 30 minutes and repeated as often as necessary.

Visiting Your Child's Doctor

If your child has a high fever, your doctor may prescribe additional fever medication. A full physical and history will often determine the type of infection and the appropriate treatment. Laboratory tests may be helpful.

Caution

Persistent fever or fever in very young children requires a full medical evaluation to determine potential sites of infection as well as the need to begin treatment

Convulsions associated with fever may just be "febrile seizures," but infection of the nervous system must often be excluded

Fever Medicine Dosage by Age*

	0–3 mo	4–11 mo	12–23 mo	2–3 yr	4–5 yr	6–8 yr	9–10 yr	11–12 yr
Acetaminophen drops (80 mg/0.8 ml)	0.4 ml	0.8 ml	1.2 ml	1.6 ml	2.4 ml			
Acetaminophen elixir (160 mg/tsp.)		½ tsp	¾ tsp	1 tsp	1½ tsp	2 tsp	2½ tsp	
Chewable tablet acetaminophen or aspirin (80 mg)			1½	2	3	4	5	6
Junior swallowable tablet (160 mg)				1	1½	2	2½	3
Adult tablet acetaminophen or aspirin (325 mg)						1	1	1½

*Your physician may recommend a higher dosage of 15 mg/kg/dose every 4–6 hours.

Headache

Headache is a common problem in adolescents and adults; children under five years rarely have headaches without an underlying illness. (See also Chap. 34.)

What to Look for

In younger children, a headache may accompany common infections such as sore throat, earache, dental abcess or sinus problems. With viral infections, muscle ache and fever often accompany the headache. Accompanying fever and neck stiffness may indicate meningitis.

In older children and adolescents, stress and tension are probably the most common causes of headaches accompanied by muscle spasms of the neck and head. The pain often worsens late in the day and may be constant, constricting or throbbing.

Throbbing, one-sided headaches are generally migraines. They have a relatively rapid onset and in many patients cause severe pain with nausea, vomiting, belly pain and eye problems. Another family member may have similar types of headaches.

Convulsions or head trauma may precede the onset. Carbon monoxide poisoning due to exposure from an unvented furnace, fire, etc., may produce headaches. Impaired vision is rarely a cause.

When to Call Your Child's Doctor

CALL IMMEDIATELY IF:

Severe, persistent pain
Stiff neck
Marked behavioral change with irritability or sleepiness
Unequal pupils
Evidence of problems including confusion, impaired speech or vision or recurrent vomiting
Traumatic head injury
Child under five years old

CALL WITHIN A FEW HOURS IF:

Persistent headache lasts longer than 48 to 72 hours
Fever without any other symptoms
Wakes child up from sleep or lasts for more than 24 hours

CALL FOR AN APPOINTMENT IF:

Recurrent headaches
Problems with friends, family or school

What You Can Do

The main goal of treatment of minor headaches is to try to minimize the pain and return to normal function. Initiate treatment as recommended by your physician.

Stress is the most common cause of headaches. Treatment may include rest, massage and counseling to reorient priorities.

Caution

Headaches in infants require evaluation to determine contributing factors.

Kidney or Bladder Infection (Urinary Tract Infections or UTIs)

Infections of the urinary tract may involve the kidney or the bladder. They are more common in girls. (See also Chap. 40.)

What to Look for

Urinary tract infections commonly cause painful (burning), frequent or bloody urination. Children may also have belly and back pain, fever, chills, nausea, vomiting and a general sense of weakness and malaise.

Girls may pass small amounts of urine or have a sense of burning on urination because of irritation, not infection. This can be due to bubble baths, trauma, masturbation or incorrect wiping (correct wiping is from front to back). Girls may have a vaginal discharge.

Blood in the urine may indicate a problem with the kidney not caused by infection.

Toilet-trained younger children may resume bed-wetting, usually in response to a new or increasing stress rather than infection.

When to Call Your Child's Doctor

CALL IMMEDIATELY IF:

Severe abdominal or back pain
High fever or chills
Blood in urine
Unable to pass urine
Swollen eyes, weight increase, headaches or decreased urination

CALL WITHIN A FEW HOURS IF:

Painful burning or frequent urination
Previous problems with urinary tract infections
Pain and other symptoms do not improve within 48 hours of beginning antibiotics
Medicines not tolerated

CALL FOR AN APPOINTMENT IF:

Recent onset of bed-wetting in child without other symptoms

What You Can Do

In girls, irritation commonly causes burning and frequent urination and may quickly be resolved by soaking in a tub of clean water with one-half cup of vinegar (without soap) for about 20 minutes. Repeat for a few days. To prevent the recurrence of the problem, use bubble bath and soap sparingly, if at all. Often, to resolve the problem, showers should be substituted for baths. Encourage wiping from front to back, and use white cotton underpants. Avoid constipation. If there are any other symptoms or an infection is possible, see your doctor.

After evaluation and prescription of antibiotics by your doctor, treat the infection at home. Give medicines for the entire prescribed course. Even when your child is feeling better, he/she may still have the infection. Follow-up visits are necessary to prevent or monitor recurrences.

Visiting Your Child's Doctor

Your doctor will examine your child for abdominal and back pain and will evaluate the genital area for irritation.

Your doctor will do a microscopic examination of a urine specimen and, if necessary, a culture. For younger children, you may use a bag to collect the urine. For older children, your doctor will need a clean sample. To obtain a clean sample from girls, wash the genital area several times with warm water and cotton. While your child is sitting on a toilet with her legs spread, have her urinate and collect some urine midstream (i.e., not at the beginning or end of the stream). Boys should similarly have midstream urine collected. If done at home, keep the specimen refrigerated in a sterile jar until your doctor's visit.

If your child has an infection, your doctor will begin antibiotics and will make arrangements for follow-up.

If no infection is present, irritation is likely and preventive steps noted above will be reviewed.

Bed-wetting may require visits to your doctor to develop an understanding of the contributing factors.

Mumps

Mumps is a viral infection of the salivary glands. There is an excellent vaccine against it. The period between exposure and illness (incubation period) is about 14 to 21 days. Children are infectious until the parotid gland swelling disappears.

What to Look for

Children have swelling of the salivary glands, most commonly the parotid gland located just in front of and below the ears. Chewing lemons or pickles make the pain worse. A low-grade fever and headache may accompany swelling. There is no rash.

Problems may include swelling and pain of the testicles as well as inflammation of the brain or pancreas.

When to Call Your Child's Doctor

CALL IMMEDIATELY IF:

Convulsions, sleepiness

CALL WITHIN A FEW HOURS IF:

Pain or swelling of testicle(s)
Abdominal pain or vomiting
Swollen lymph nodes ("glands") of the neck

What You Can Do

Reduce discomfort with acetaminophen. Encourage fluids and avoid sour substances and citrus fruits. If testicular pain develops, rest, support and pain medicines are usually adequate. Check to be certain that your other children are immunized.

Visiting Your Child's Doctor

After identifying the illness as mumps (as opposed to swollen lymph nodes), your doctor will examine your child for complications and will suggest specific measures, if necessary.

Poisoning

Most accidental poisoning occurs in children who are under five years old. In those under one year, poisoning is usually due to parental mistake in giving medicines. Older children are adventuresome and curious, sporadically experimenting with any products and medications they may find.

What You Can Do

Children who ingest either potentially dangerous substances or excessive amounts of normally safe products require careful examination.

Make sure your child is acting and breathing normally. Flush exposed area or induce vomiting.

Skin exposed to acids, caustics or insecticides should be flooded with water and washed with soap. Remove all contaminated clothing.

Eyes exposed to acids or caustics should be washed immediately for 15 to 20 minutes before taking your child to your doctor. Hold your child's head under running water in a sink or shower or pour water into the eye from a pitcher or a glass.

Taken by mouth: Vomiting should be induced using syrup of ipecac in children over six months of age in the following amounts:

Six to 12-month-old	Give two teaspoons
One to 12-year-old	Give three teaspoons (one-half ounce)
Over 12 years	Give six teaspoons (one ounce)

It is often valuable to call your poison-control center before giving syrup of ipecac, since the poisoning may not be serious and may require no therapy.

If syrup of ipecac is given, encourage your child to drink water or clear liquids and to walk around, if possible. Give another dose of syrup of ipecac if your child does not vomit after 20 minutes. If necessary, a throat stick, spoon or finger at the back of the throat may be useful.

DO NOT USE syrup of ipecac if your child has taken acid or caustics such as strong household cleaners, lye, strong bleach, etc. Give your child water or milk to dilute the substance and call your doctor or poison center to get immediate medical attention.

DO NOT USE syrup of ipecac if your child is sleepy or unresponsive.

Call your regional poison control center! This is probably the quickest place to receive advice on the nature of the substance your child has taken and the severity of the poisoning. You should review your plans with the center and arrange for your doctor or the nearest emergency department to see your child.

Take your child to a hospital or to a doctor!

In most cases your child should be seen by your doctor or an emergency department unless the poison control center says the ingested substance(s) was not toxic or dangerous. To permit an accurate identification, take the container with the medication or substance ingested with you.

Dangerous household substances, such as medications, dishwasher soap, cleaning supplies, drain-cleaning crystals or liquids, paints and thinners, automobile products and garden sprays, must be put away in locked cabinets. Always keep medications in child-proof containers! Be particularly watchful during periods of disruptions such as moving, travel, visitors, etc. Often grandparents have medications in a container, purse or piece of baggage that is not child-proof.

Have syrup of ipecac in the house for emergencies.

Rashes

Rashes in children come in many sizes, colors and shapes. It is hard to distinguish different types of skin problems; the following list may help sort out some of the more common ones:

Rashes that are Red without Bumps:

Measles (Rubeola)
Rubella (German or three-day measles)
Roseola
Scarlet fever
Drug (ampicillin) rash
Erythema infectiosum (Fifth disease)
"Viral rash"

Rashes that are Red with Bumps:

Acne
Candidiasis (monila diaper rash)
Contact dermatitis
Diaper rash
Eczema
Hives
Impetigo
Insect bite
Ringworm

Rashes with Blisters (fluid-filled):

Chicken pox (Varicella)
Herpes zoster
Impetigo, bullous
Insect bite
Scabies

Rashes that are purple or red without blanching (i.e., when the skin is pulled tight between two fingers, rash still appears red or purple), these are virtually always emergencies.

(See also Chap. 13.)

When to Call Your Child's Doctor

If you are uncertain what kind of rash your child has or if there are problems.

CALL IMMEDIATELY IF:

Purple, red or blood-like without blanching
Burn-like
Red, blue or tender to the touch
Red-streaking
Pustular

CALL WITHIN A FEW HOURS IF:

Skin is itchy
Child looks sick
Fever lasts over 24 hours
Rash related to medications
Pustules present with red or cola-colored urine

If the rash concerns you, your child appears to be sick or the rash persists, you should call your doctor because identifying rashes is difficult.

Rash—Chicken Pox (Varicella)

Chicken pox is an infection caused by a virus. The time between exposure to someone with chicken pox and the beginning of the illness (incubation period) is 14 to 21 days. Children are infectious from one day before the rash appears until the blisters dry and crust over (seven days). It spreads very easily.

What to Look for

RASH

Look for a sudden onset of flat, red spots that become small, raised bumps and finally small blisters surrounded by a red area. The rash is primarily on the trunk and is very itchy, tending to appear in groups of lesions in different stages. After the blisters break, they scab over and form a crust. Some children have only a few lesions while others are totally covered.

OTHER

Preceding the rash, there are usually no symptoms except for an occasional fever which may persist during the illness. Lesions may become infected, producing impetigo. Rarely, patients may develop a lung infection or have impaired responsiveness.

When to Call Your Child's Doctor

CALL IMMEDIATELY IF:

Marked toxicity or your child looks very ill
Rapid or difficult breathing
Convulsion, sleepiness or severe headache
Underlying disease in your child

CALL WITHIN A FEW HOURS IF:

Lesions get red, warm, tender or drain pus
Your newborn is exposed to chicken pox

What You Can Do

Keep your child comfortable. Give baking soda baths (one-half cup in tub) to soothe. Use Calamine lotion on the skin. Cut fingernails to minimize scratching. If your child is having trouble drinking, have him/her gargle with salt water. If the throat is still sore, have your child gargle with an antacid like Mylanta or Maalox to coat the mouth.

Start antihistamines, such as Benadryl, for severe itching. Do not use aspirin. Keep your child out of day care or school until the blisters crust over.

Visiting Your Child's Doctor

Rarely is a visit required unless there are specific, worrisome problems.

Rash – Contact Dermatitis

Skin irritants can cause rashes. Typical substances include alkali, detergents, plants (poison ivy and poison oak), medicine put on the skin, as well as shoes, nickel and cosmetics.

What to Look for

The skin is red and swollen; blisters and crusts may form. The distribution of the rash follows the pattern of contact.

When to Call Your Child's Doctor

CALL WITHIN A FEW HOURS IF:

Weepy, blistery lesion with swelling

What You Can Do

No therapy is usually necessary except for avoiding the irritating substance. If the irritation is extensive, hydration of the skin may help. After baths, apply a mild lotion, such as Eucerin or Nivea, before drying your child off. Another alternative is to apply towels or cloths moistened with warm water to weeping areas to clear up the involved region.

If the problem is particularly bothersome, applying steroid cream (hydrocortisone) to the area may hasten healing.

Avoid future contact with the offending substance.

Visiting Your Child's Doctor

If the problem is severe, your doctor may prescribe special medicine to decrease the swelling and irritation.

Rash – Diaper Dermatitis and Candidiasis

Prolonged contact between skin and urine or stool in the diaper area produces irritation and dampness. This may lead to additional irritation from *Candida*.

What to Look for

The diaper area is red, with small blisters or areas of minor ulcer. If small, red areas with bumps are present, often in areas of creases appearing as "kissing lesions," the child also has *monilia* which is due to an infection of *Candida*. Many children with monilia also have red areas with white patches on the inside of the mouth, which is known as *thrush*.

When to Call Your Child's Doctor

CALL FOR AN APPOINTMENT IF:

No improvement with home treatment
Red areas with bumps along creases

What You Can Do

Keep the diaper area clean by changing diapers frequently and cleaning the area each time using warm water. Occasionally, mild soaps will help such as Neutrogena, Basis, Lowila or Cetaphil.

Leave your child without a diaper as much as possible, particularly during naps. Fasten diapers loosely. If you use cloth diapers, double-rinse them. Do not use plastic pants. If you use disposable diapers, punch a few holes in the plastic liner. Sometimes children do better with one brand of diapers rather than another. You may want to try several brands.

If there are red areas with bumps along the creases, you may need to apply special cream to the involved areas at diaper changes. If there are white areas in your child's mouth, you may give a similar oral medication by mouth that can be prescribed by your doctor.

Visiting Your Child's Doctor

Only rarely do children with a diaper rash need to visit the doctor. If the rash is bad or difficult to treat, your doctor can prescribe special medication to hasten healing.

Rash—Eczema or Atopic Dermatitis

Eczema is often present with other allergic conditions and is at least partially due to an inability to retain moisture in the skin, i.e., the skin is too dry. There may be a family history of allergies.

What to Look for

Skin is red, dry and scaly, involving areas of irritation on the body as well as the face. Involved areas are usually symmetrically distributed and become progressively red and swollen with crusting and weeping. Children usually itch. Infection with crusting and pus occurs occasionally.

When to Call Your Child's Doctor

CALL WITHIN A FEW HOURS IF:

Marked redness, crusting or weepy lesions
Infection with crusting or pus

CALL FOR AN APPOINTMENT IF:

No response to therapy

What You Can Do

In mild disease without significant weeping or crusting, try to hydrate the skin. Bathe your child and then apply Eucerin lotion to involved areas without drying the skin. Do not use soap. Cetaphil lotion may be used instead. If there is a small area with marked redness, a steroid cream such as hydrocortisone may be used for one to two days.

Moderate problems require more active steps for two to three days. Apply a towel or cloth dampened with warm water to the involved areas. Remove, rewet and reapply towels every five minutes for a total of three treatments. Repeat three times daily. At night, bathe your child, put on damp cotton pajamas and then cover with a second, dry pair. If necessary, use a steroid cream as well as antihistamines, such as Benadryl, to reduce itching.

After the skin has improved, improve hydration with daily baths and applications of Eucerin to the wet skin without drying off your child. In mild cases, use lubricating creams such as Nivea. Do not use soap; Cetaphil lotion is a good soap substitute. Keep fingernails short.

Rash—Hives (or Urticaria)

Hives are an allergic reaction to substances such as food, medicines, insect bites, etc.

What to Look for

RASH

Red, raised lesions with marked swelling that are often itchy. They are often called "welts."

Ampicillin and amoxicillin commonly cause a rash, which may be related to an allergy but more commonly is not. The non-allergic rash consists of small bumps with a slightly red base appearing seven to 10 days after beginning the medicine. Allergic problems begin in the first four to five days.

OTHER

Difficult or rapid breathing

When to Call Your Child's Doctor

CALL IMMEDIATELY IF:

Difficult or rapid breathing

CALL WITHIN A FEW HOURS IF:

Bothersome itching

What You Can Do

If the itching is bothersome, antihistamines, such as Benadryl, may be useful. If there are associated problems, the adequacy of the airway and breathing must be assessed immediately.

It is important to exclude things that cause problems such as drugs, eggs, milk, chocolate, shellfish, cheese, nuts, pollens and insect bites.

Visiting Your Child's Doctor

A visit is only required if there is difficulty breathing. Your doctor needs to administer medications quickly to reverse the process.

Rash – Impetigo

Impetigo is a superficial infection of the skin that occurs with cuts, abrasions or irritation of the skin. It is more frequent in the summer.

What to Look for

RASH

Small, red areas quickly develop blisters and then form a honey-colored crust. They may spread. Large blisters that grow together may also appear. The face, arms, legs and areas of abrasion are most commonly involved.

OTHER

Rarely, the kidney is involved, producing a gray, cola-colored urine.

When to Call Your Child's Doctor

CALL WITHIN A FEW HOURS IF:

Blisters are crusting over
No response to medicines
Cola-colored urine

What You Can Do

Scrub and soak the involved area to try to loosen or dissolve any crusts that have formed. Antibiotics will not cure the problem unless the crusts are removed. Give all doses of medicine until the prescription is completely finished. Minimize sharing of towels, sheets, etc.

Visiting Your Child's Doctor

After making the diagnosis, your doctor will prescribe antibiotics and will give you instructions about removing crusts and keeping your child clean.

Rash – Lice

Lice are small insects that are usually found in the head and genital areas. People transmit them to other people.

What to Look for

Small, raised bumps are present in the head and genital area. "Nits" (lice eggs) may also be found in these areas. There is usually a great deal of associated itching.

When to Call Your Child's Doctor

CALL FOR AN APPOINTMENT IF:

Severe itching, particularly if no response to home management

What You Can Do

Several products are available, some without a prescription, that should kill the lice. RID and NIX are common, as is Kwell shampoo. Apply RID undiluted to the infested area, allow to remain for 10 minutes and then wash off thoroughly. Give a second treatment in seven to 10 days. For Kwell shampoo, apply to the area and work into a lather with water for four minutes and then wash thoroughly. Treat others who have a similar rash and have had contact with your child, if they are not pregnant.

You can comb out nits. Washing the hair with undiluted, warm vinegar makes this easier. If the eyebrows or lashes are involved, apply petrolatum (Vaseline) carefully to the area overnight.

Wash your child's bed linens and clothes that have been worn recently. For four days don't allow your child to wear hats and other headgear that are difficult to wash. Use antihistamines, such as Benadryl, if itching is a problem.

Visiting Your Child's Doctor

Rarely, a visit is needed to confirm the diagnosis.

Rash – Ringworm

Ringworm is a skin infection caused by a fungus.

What to Look for

The lesions start as small, round, red spots and slowly get larger with a scaly outer rim and a relatively clear center. They are most common on the face, arms, shoulders, or groin and may be itchy. Infection may develop.

When to Call Your Child's Doctor

CALL FOR AN APPOINTMENT IF:

Lesions get red, warm, tender or drain pus
Scalp or nails are involved
No improvement. Spreading after a week of medicine

What You Can Do

Purchase tinactin (or similar) cream, available without a perscription, and apply to the involved areas two times daily for up to several weeks. Continue the medicine for a week after the problem has cleared up.

Visiting Your Child's Doctor

If the lesions are not going away, your doctor will probably scrape a small sample of the scales, look at them under a microscope to confirm the diagnosis and prescribe other medicines. Infections of the scalp or nails require special medications taken for a prolonged period.

Rash—Scarlet Fever

Scarlet fever describes the combination of rash, fever and sore throat associated with streptococcal infection (Group A).

What to Look for

RASH

Small, red bumps are present, and the skin feels like sandpaper. Usually the area around the mouth is pale, and skin creases are pronounced. The rash lasts about five to seven days and then peels.

OTHER

Sore throat, swollen lymph nodes, headache, fever, and abdominal pain may all occur.

When to Call Your Child's Doctor

CALL WITHIN A FEW HOURS IF:

Small, red bumps; sandpapery skin; pale mouth area; pronounced skin creases
Sore throat, fever, swollen lymph nodes, headache or belly pain

What You Can Do

Scarlet fever is no more serious than any strep throat. In the older child, throat lozenges or hard candy, especially butterscotch, are soothing to the throat. Use honey for young children over one year old. Acetaminophen is good for relieving pain. Some children respond well to gargling warm water.

Your doctor will prescribe antibiotics. Give as indicated until the entire prescription is taken. Children are contagious for 24 hours after starting the medicine.

Visiting Your Child's Doctor

After doing a complete examination to confirm the diagnosis, your physician will usually do a throat culture and prescribe medicine to treat the infection. Sometimes your doctor will do a throat culture at the end of treatment.

Sore Throat

Sore throats are common in children, often with other complaints related to a streptococcal or viral infection. (See also Chap. 17.)

What to Look for

Sore throats often cause painful swallowing with fever, big lymph nodes ("glands") in the neck, headache and belly pain. Your child may complain of difficulty eating and swallowing or be resistant to drinking and eating.

Streptococcal infections are difficult to differentiate from viral infections without a throat culture but more commonly have associated fever, white pus on the tonsils, tender and enlarged lymph nodes and marked difficulty swallowing. Streptococcal infections may also cause a sandpapery fine rash (scarlet fever) with accentuation of the creases at joints.

More serious infections produce a painful throat. Rarely, they may cause drooling or marked difficulty with swallowing, breathing or moving the jaw. "Fever" or canker sores produce pain on swallowing as do dental cavities.

When to Call Your Child's Doctor

CALL IMMEDIATELY IF:

Severe difficulty swallowing
Difficulty breathing or any drooling
Pain or limitation of jaw movement
Extreme pain

CALL WITHIN A FEW HOURS (CULTURE USUALLY INDICATED) IF:

Fever, white pus on tonsils, tender lymph nodes or sandpapery fine rash
Belly pain
Headache

CALL FOR AN APPOINTMENT IF:

Exposure to streptococcus at home or school with any symptoms at present
Frequent sore throats
Sore throat present over 48 hours

What You Can Do

Before starting home treatment, arrange for your child to see your doctor if indicated. Home treatment in older children may include throat lozenges or hard candy, especially butterscotch, to soothe the throat. Use honey for children over one year old. Acetaminophen (Tylenol, Tempra, etc.) is good for relieving the pain. Some children respond well to gargling with warm water.

Visiting Your Child's Doctor

Your doctor will usually do a 24-hour streptococcal culture (quick tests in the office are often available) if your child has symptoms that may be caused by a strep infection. Cultures are not necessary for exposed but healthy children.

If your child's culture is positive, your doctor will start antibiotics. Usually your child will feel better in one to two days. Give the medicines as directed for the entire 10-day course; not finishing the total treatment can cause kidney or heart irritation. Children are contagious for 24 hours after starting treatment but may return to school or day care after this period.

If the culture is negative, discontinue antibiotics and discard them.

Sudden Infant Death Syndrome

Sudden infant death syndrome (SIDS) is a devastating event whereby a child dies unexpectedly of an unexplained cause. Although children up to one year old may suffer SIDS, the majority of deaths occur between two and four months of age. Many SIDS victims have recently had a cold, cough, fever, vomiting or diarrhea. (See also Chap. 43.)

What to Look for

Commonly, children will experience a near-SIDS episode, whereby they briefly stop breathing but then quickly resume, often in response to your early resuscitative efforts. Immediate help can save these children. Begin CPR immediately. If SIDS has taken place, your child will not be breathing and his/her heart will not be beating. Immediate action is required to restore lung and heart activity. Begin CPR immediately.

When to Call Your Child's Doctor

CALL IMMEDIATELY (CALL 911):

In all cases or if your child is not breathing

What You Can Do

Begin life support for your children. Children who have had a near-SIDS episode can be resuscitated; your actions must be aggressive and directed towards the lungs and heart.

You can learn cardiopulmonary resuscitation through courses offered by the American Red Cross.

Arrange immediate transfer to the nearest emergency center.

Visiting Your Child's Doctor

To provide optimal care, your child will be taken to the nearest emergency department. Steps to support your child's airway will often have been completed; early assessment will focus on deciding how much potential injury has occurred.

If full resuscitation is indicated, the hospital staff will mobilize its resources and initiate a number of procedures. You will see a host of physicians and assistants working toward one goal–saving your child.

Vomiting

Gastroenteritis or "stomach flu" usually causes vomiting. Minimal spitting up or regurgitation may be normal in infants and decreases as your child gets older. It becomes a problem if it suddenly increases in amount or frequency. (See also Chap. 26.)

What to Look for

Vomiting is often accompanied by nausea, fever, and diarrhea from either an irritation or an infection of the intestines. Changing the diet often improves this. Additional symptoms imply other problems. Watch for green, bloody or "coffee ground" vomitus; swelling of the abdomen or marked changes in behavior.

Infections of the ear, urinary tract and brain can cause vomiting, usually without diarrhea. Accidental poisoning with lead or excessive aspirin can cause vomiting with blood. After a head injury, vomiting can occur immediately and become problematic if it continues. Vomiting after injury to the belly or swallowing a foreign body can mean there is some blockage.

Some neonates and infants spit up a great deal of vomit occasionally. *Chalasia* results from the muscle between the stomach and food pipe being too relaxed and allowing food from the stomach to come back into the mouth, often within 30 to 45 minutes of feeding. It is common in newborns; as long as your infant is doing well, it is an inconvenience rather than something to be concerned about.

Spitting up may also be caused by feeding problems and techniques.

Dehydration (loss of water) may develop.

When to Call Your Child's Doctor

CALL IMMEDIATELY IF:

Vomitus has blood
Severe or prolonged (more than two hours) abdominal pain
Belly or head injury
Poisoning
Possible foreign body
Behavioral changes causing irritability or listlessness
Dehydration with decreased urination, less moisture in diapers, no tears, rapid breathing, irritability or sleepiness

CALL WITHIN A FEW HOURS IF:

Vomiting for more than 24 hours
Vomiting without diarrhea
Child is routinely taking medications that may contribute to vomiting
Painful, frequent or bloody urination
Ear pain

CALL FOR AN APPOINTMENT IF:

Recurrent problem

What You Can Do

Avoid solids for six to eight hours. Small feedings usually work, often starting with tablespoon amounts of clear liquids. These fluids may include Pedialyte or Lytren for the infant, popsicles, ice chips and room-temperature, defizzed soda in older children. Slowly increase the amount over six to eight hours. After this period without vomiting, slowly expand the diet to include toast, dry crackers, clear soup, broth, etc.

Infants with chalasia usually respond to careful attention to feeding techniques. Keep your child in an upright position during feeding. It is often helpful to keep your child upright in an infant chair during the 30 to 45 minutes following feeding. Feed your baby frequently with small amounts and burp often. Use formula or milk thickened with small amounts of dry cereal.

A foreign body in the intestines does not necessarily mean that there is a blockage. If no other problem exists and your doctor doesn't think the object is stuck, watch your child's stool for passage.

Cuts and Scrapes

Cuts and scrapes are common for children and usually involve a minor, superficial injury.

What to Look for

Often, cuts and scratches only need to be cleansed and washed; at other times, they need stitching (suturing) and additional treatment. Look for the following in determining if medical treatment is needed:

DEPTH OF THE WOUND

The depth of the wound determines the involvement of internal structures such as muscle, tendons, blood vessels and nerves. Injury that is limited to the skin and fatty tissue beneath may require only cleansing and suturing; injury to other tissues requires repair before suturing.

Puncture wounds are difficult to evaluate; those on the extremities rarely cause much deep injury. Active bleeding, numbness or a foreign body left in the wound will probably need exploration.

SIZE OF THE WOUND

Larger wounds usually require suturing to hold the edges together and to minimize scarring. Abrasions and scratches usually require cleaning.

LOCATION OF THE WOUND

It is important to minimize scarring following cuts and abrasions on the face. Stitching the face is more time consuming and requires more meticulous care than other areas. Wounds on the hands or feet often involve deeper sutures, while other areas, such as the genital region, are difficult to care for without training.

MECHANISM OF INJURY

Accidents involving motor vehicles or those suggesting the possibility of bad injuries to many parts of the body demand a full examination of your child.

If your child's arm is caught in a wringer-like device, the injury may appear minor on the surface but may involve significant injury to the arm tissues.

If a body part such as a finger or toe is accidentally amputated, place it in a clean plastic bag and place the bag in iced water. If no bag is available, place the body part in a clean cloth. Do not immerse in water or ice directly.

Poorly explained injuries may indicate abuse. They require evaluation.

Electrical or chemical injuries require medical assessment.

TETANUS STATUS

Children require immunization for protection from tetanus. Children with a major injury who have completed their initial shot schedule need an additional immunization if it has been more than five years since their last tetanus shot. Children with a minor injury need an additional immunization if it has been more than 10 years since their last tetanus shot. Obviously if they are behind on immunizations, this may be a good opportunity to update tetanus shots.

INFECTION

After several days, wounds may become infected, developing warmth, redness and tenderness around the area, and occasionally draining pus. Any infections should be seen by your child's doctor.

When to Call Your Child's Doctor

CALL IMMEDIATELY IF:

Possibility of major injury from a motor vehicle or other worrisome mechanism

Bleeding despite continuous pressure
Deep or large cut
Possible involvement of muscle, tendon, nerve or blood vessel
Cut on face or hand
Redness, tenderness, warmth or pus around wound
Wringer-type or unexplained injury
Cut or abrasion on head with any change in behavior or state of alertness

CALL WITHIN A FEW HOURS IF:

Minor cut with skin split open, i.e., needs sutures
Abrasion on face, hand, feet, genital region or large area
Any question about the need for tetanus immunization

What You Can Do

Initially, put direct pressure on the wound for at least 15 minutes with a washcloth, towel or other cloth. If the initial dressing becomes soaked with blood, place additional dressings on the injury while maintaining pressure. Keep the injured area elevated at a level above the heart. After bleeding has stopped, wash the area with water (and soap, if available). Apply ice to the area to reduce swelling. Rinse well and be certain that there is no dirt, glass or other foreign material present.

Once bleeding has stopped, examine the wound more fully. If your doctor does not need to see it, make certain that it is clean. Any loose skin can be cut off with clean scissors. Wounds that appear to need professional evaluation should be seen without delay. If suturing is appropriate, your doctor will want to do it within several hours to reduce the risk of infection. After too long a period of time, suturing may not be possible.

If the cut is small, leave it exposed. Apply a nonstick dressing of gauze to a larger wound. Minor wounds that do not need sutures may benefit from bringing the edges together; do this by holding them together with "butterfly" bandages or by cutting a bandage or tape into small pieces to bridge the gap.

Soak puncture wounds in water and soap for a minimum of 10 to 15 minutes. These are not usually sutured. See your doctor for an in-depth evaluation if there is active, ongoing bleeding, numbness or pain.

Following the visit to your doctor, mild bleeding and discomfort may occur as the numbing medicine wears off. Follow specific instructions, but in general, keep the wound clean and dry for two days. You may wash it gently with soap and water. Dressings should generally be changed every day. If sutures have been placed, gently soak the area with water or peroxide one to two days before the sutures are to be removed to reduce scabs. This may make removal of sutures easier. Return to your doctor as directed to have sutures removed.

Special circumstances that may occasionally require a visit to your doctor:

Blood collections may occur **under the fingernail or toenail** after a finger or toe has been smashed with a hammer or other hard object. If the pain is severe, relieve it by making a hole in the fingernail. Open a paper clip and heat one end with a candle, cigarette lighter or fire. When the tip is red hot, touch it quickly to the nail and melt through the nail leaving a small hole and draining the blood.

Fishhooks can become embedded in your child's skin. Hook a thread around the curve of the hook. Push down on the hook's eye and shank to disengage the barb and then align the string with the long axis of the shank. Pull gently. If unsuccessful, the hook can be pushed all the way through and the barb cut off.

Remove a ring on a swollen finger by alternating five-minute intervals of soaking the finger in cold water and elevating it. Continue for a total of 30 minutes. Apply oil (mineral or cooking) to the finger. Another approach is to place a string under the ring and wrap it in loops around the finger from the end of the finger closest to palm proceeding to the tip. The loops should be close and firm enough to depress and shrink the flesh. Pull the palm end of the string back toward the tip of the finger and tug slowly while pulling the ring off as the string unwinds. The ring may also be cut off with a ring cutter.

Visiting Your Child's Doctor

Your doctor will examine your child to determine the extent of injury and the involvement of any internal structures. Then your doctor will use numbing medicine to reduce any discomfort before cleansing and reexploring the wound. If internal structures are injured, your doctor will repair them before suturing the skin.

Your child may require a tetanus immunization.

Often, your doctor may want to check the wound in a few days to be certain that it is healing well and that no infection develops.

Facial sutures will be removed in three or five days, while those in other areas will be left in longer.

Caution

Your doctor should see any cut or scrape that may involve deeper tissues or may require suturing.

Facial injuries

A number of injuries may occur to the face including damage to the eyes or mouth.

What to Look for

Eye injuries are common. Normal vision is a good indicator that the injury is probably not severe. Eye pain may occur from scratches on the eye surface. Blunt trauma with an object small enough to fit within the eye rim may cause blood in the front of the eye, often associated with a loss of vision.

Dental injuries occur from blows to the teeth from falls, sports or fights. Determine if the teeth involved are primary (baby) or permanent. Injuries can cause teeth to become tender, sensitive to cold or touch, loose, cracked, missing or displaced. Bleeding can occur at the margin of the gums and the teeth. A dentist should see such problems immediately if a permanent tooth is involved and promptly if only primary teeth are injured.

Mouth injuries are usually minor but may produce problems if not identified and cared for at an early stage. Small cuts on the inside of the mouth or on the tongue usually heal but may need suturing if they are large or deep. Children who fall with pencils or sticks in their mouths may puncture or otherwise injure internal structures and increase the risk of infection.

When to Call Your Child's Doctor

CALL IMMEDIATELY IF:

Loss or blurring of vision
Blood in the front part of the eye
Injury to a permanent tooth
Difficulty breathing through one or both nostrils
Nosebleed continuing despite 10 minutes of continuous pressure

CALL WITHIN A FEW HOURS IF:

Eye pain
Injured primary tooth
Displacement of nose
Fall with a pencil or stick in the mouth
Explanation does not explain injury

What You Can Do

Facial injuries often accompany other trauma. If there are other injuries, they are usually taken care of first. It is essential to make certain that the airway is clear and that breathing is adequate.

If there is an **eye injury**, check vision. If it is partially or totally impaired or there is eye pain, decide where to go for help. Patch the eye with the eyelid closed with a cloth or gauze until it can be examined to prevent further damage.

If a **tooth** is loose, try to reposition it with gentle pressure. Once in position, hold for five to 10 minutes. If a permanent tooth is lost, hold the tooth carefully by the crown (the part that is normally exposed) and wash gently with water to get rid of foreign material. Insert the tooth into the socket as soon as possible. If you cannot replace the tooth in its normal position, place the tooth under your child's or your tongue to bathe in saliva or place it in room-temperature milk while taking your child to the dentist. For a tooth to be successfully reimplanted, it should be done within one to two hours. The sooner the better!

Nosebleeds usually respond to compression of the soft and bony part of the nose, pressing downward toward the cheeks with the thumb and forefinger for a minimum of 10 minutes.

If there is a cut in the **mouth**, have your child rinse it. Encourage clear liquids over the next 12 hours. Ice or Popsicles may be useful.

If there is any evidence of **neck pain** or tenderness, try to lie your child down and keep his/her head still. Place your child on a board and tape the head facing straight up. Use filler material, such as towels or clothes on both sides of the head. Usually call emergency vehicle (911) to arrange transport to the hospital.

Head Injury

Children are constantly bumping their heads or, less commonly, falling or being hit by some moving object. Usually no problems develop, but your child must be watched to be sure no complications develop.

What to Look for

The circumstances of the accident are important. The type of injury is determined by whether the accident was the result of a direct blow from a strong force, a serious fall or an accident involving a moving vehicle. Children may lose consciousness immediately following such an injury or have a period of relatively normal behavior followed by problems. Following head trauma, children may have a loss of memory or be disoriented or dizzy. They may develop visual problems, vomiting, nausea, headache, neck pain or convulsions.

Determine immediately if your child has any neck pain.

When to Call Your Child's Doctor

CALL IMMEDIATELY IF:

Injury involves a large force, a serious fall or a motor vehicle
Decreased consciousness immediately or soon thereafter. Does not know name, date, location
Irregular breathing or pulse
Loss of consciousness for more than five seconds
Increased sleepiness or drowsiness, or inability to waken patient from sleep
Change in equality of pupils (i.e., the black centers of the eyes become unequal in size), blurred vision, peculiar movements of the eyes or difficulty in focusing
Stumbling, unusual weakness, problem using arms or legs, or change in normal gait or crawl
Personality or behavior change, such as increasing irritability, confusion, restlessness or inability to concentrate
Persistent vomiting (more than three times)
Blood or fluid drainage from nose or ears
Black eyes or brusing behind ears immediately following injury
Convulsions or seizures
Neck pain
Large cut, persistent bleeding or deformity of head

CALL WITHIN A FEW HOURS IF:

Cut requiring suturing but without order problems
Headache worsening
Explanation does not adequately explain injury

What You Can Do

Make certain that your child's breathing is adequate and that no other problems exist. Place a cold cloth on the point of impact to reduce swelling. Watch your child for changes in behavior or alertness for at least a day following the accident. Examine your child every two to four hours to be certain that he/she is improving. Continue to monitor the pupils (black spot in the center of the eye), level of consciousness and communication skills. Awaken as necessary.

Wash and clean any cuts and scrapes after bleeding has stopped. Large or deep cuts may need stitches.

Give aspirin or acetaminophen for pain. Stronger medicines will not usually be given because of the importance of watching your child's behavior and alertness over the next day.

Limit activities and restrict to a light diet.

If there is neck pain or tenderness, don't allow your child to move around. Gently position your hands on the sides of his/her head until you can place your child carefully on a board and tape the head facing straight up from the board. Use filler material (such as towels or clothes) on either side of the head to keep it from moving.

Caution

All patients with bad head injuries or worrisome findings need evaluation and observation.

All children with neck pain or tenderness following injury should have their head and neck restrained to prevent movement until the neck injury can be evaluated.

Neck Pain and Swelling

Pain or swelling of the neck commonly occurs with infection or injury to the neck.

What to Look for

Children complaining of neck pain or swelling usually have swollen lymph nodes ("glands") due to a sore throat or other infection of the airway. Streptococcal infection is a common cause, particularly when the lymph nodes are tender with overlying redness of the skin.

Small nodes in the back of the head, behind the ears and in the neck region are common in children. Nodes often enlarge in response to a small cut, abrasion or infection. This can occur not only with nodes in the neck but in other areas such as the groin, armpit or elbow.

A high fever, difficulty touching the chin to the chest, marked behavioral changes, discomfort with swallowing, difficulty breathing or drooling may indicate more serious infection.

An injury with neck pain, any loss of sensation or strength, or pains shooting into the arm requires immobilization of the neck. These symptoms commonly follow accidents in automobiles or on trampolines. Do not move your child until it can be done safely, usually using a hard board and taping the head with the assistance of ambulance personnel.

In infancy, pressure on the neck during delivery often produces bleeding in the muscle with swelling and pain on movement. When older children pull a neck muscle, they develop a stiff neck known as torticollis or wry neck.

When to Call Your Child's Doctor

CALL IMMEDIATELY IF:

Neck trauma (do not move without immobilization). Usually call 911
High fever, difficulty touching chin to chest or behavioral change
Drooling or difficulty breathing
Discomfort with swallowing
Stiff neck without tenderness
Extreme pain

CALL WITHIN A FEW HOURS IF:

Lymph nodes ("glands") are tender or larger than three inches or if overlying skin is red
Fever over 102°F (39°C) or any elevated temperature lasting longer than 24 hours
Sore throat or ear pain
Pain lasting more than 48 hours

What You Can Do

Treat muscle spasm or injury with heating pads and massage combined with mild pain-relief muscle-relaxation medication in older children. Recurrent problems in an older child may require specific physical therapy.

Most large nodes caused by infections, particularly when they are tender with overlying redness, are due to streptococcus and respond to antibiotics. Use acetaminophen (Tylenol, Tempra, etc.) for fever control. The nodes commonly become non-tender after 24 to 36 hours. They may remain large for weeks or months.

Immediately immobilize a traumatized or injured child who has neck pain. Logroll (DO NOT LIFT) your child onto a stiff board and tape his/her head down. Keep your child calm by offering reassurance, talking and stroking his/her head.

Visiting Your Child's Doctor

After careful examination of the neck, your doctor will decide if the problem is injury or infection. Different types of infection require different treatments, often combined with antibiotics. Your doctor may exclude serious infections by using special tests.

If the pain is due to trauma with muscle spasm, the neck, collarbone or shoulder may require X-ray studies. If there is no bone damage, your doctor may make suggestions for relieving your child's discomfort.

Caution

A child with a nontender stiff neck, difficulty breathing, or high fever often has a serious infection requiring immediate evaluation

Never move a child with neck trauma or injury and neck pain until it can be done safely

Sprains and Broken Bones

Children are frequently involved in accidents that produce pain, swelling and tenderness of their arms, legs, hands or feet. Although these accidents usually cause only bruises or sprains, broken bones can occur. The greater the force involved, the more likely there is to be a fracture. Children's bones are more easily injured than adults' but heal more rapidly.

What to Look for

When trying to determine what kind of injuries there are, it helps to find out how the accident happened. The nature of the injury should conform to the mechanism.

Tenderness, swelling and bruising may be present over the painful area. On the basis of physical examination alone, it is very difficult to be certain that a bone is not broken. Particular problems may arise if the area is cold, blue or numb or looks deformed, with or without the bone exposed. Children are often unwilling to bear weight or make normal movements with an injured extremity.

When to Call Your Child's Doctor

CALL IMMEDIATELY IF:

Limb or joint is deformed or shortened
Limb is cold, blue or numb
Extreme pain
Pelvis, hip or thigh is tender
Child is pale, sweaty or dizzy (may worsen when sits or stands)
After casting is applied, severe pain or pressure within the cast, increasing blueness or coldness, excessive swelling or decreased motion of the fingers or toes that are involved

CALL WITHIN A FEW HOURS IF:

Unable to bear weight
Decreased use, movement or function of limb
Moderate pain
Marked swelling
Bleeding or laceration
Injury to elbow with marked swelling
Mechanism does not explain injury

CALL FOR AN APPOINTMENT IF:

Persistent pain beyond 48 hours
Reduced mobility of limb in days and weeks following injury

What You Can Do

Apply ice to involved area and keep elevated to lessen pain and swelling. Gently touch to determine how much swelling, pain and deformity are present. Compare the injured area with the same region on the other limb. If there is bleeding, apply pressure.

In most cases, take your child for evaluation. It is often useful to explain to children what may happen. A brief discussion about X-rays may be reassuring. (There is no pain if they hold still; it's like taking a picture.) Arrange immediate assessment if there is a deformity or evidence of poor circulation (blue, cool or numb). Deformed limbs, especially if the bone is visible, should be moved as little as possible. Rolled-up magazines or newspapers may serve as a temporary splint. Splint the joints above and below the involved area.

If there is only a sprain, elevate the limb and apply ice packs for the first 24 hours. Rest is essential, although it is useful to wiggle the finger or toes periodically. An elastic bandage and crutches restrict movement and prevent weight bearing or use. Slings are useful for shoulder problems.

Keep the cast dry (unless a Fiberglass cast is used). Do not place foreign objects under the cast or pull the padding out. If there is severe pain or pressure within the cast, increasing coolness or blueness of the fingers or toes, your doctor may need to apply a new cast.

Once a cast or bandage is removed, your child will feel weak, but should gradually increase activity.

Visiting Your Child's Doctor

Your doctor will determine the extent of the bone injury and if there is nerve or blood vessel damage. An X-ray will determine if there is a fracture. If there is no fracture, your doctor may recommend rest for the joint using a combination of elastic bandage, sling, crutches or splint.

Specific problems are very common in children:

Broken clavicle (collarbone) commonly occurs from falls or blows to the shoulder. Children may complain of pain over the collarbone and refuse to use their arm. A special splint ("figure of 8") keeps the shoulders straight. Collarbone fractures heal well.

Pulling an infant's arm may produce a **nursemaid's elbow**. The child will not use the arm because of pain at the elbow. If there are no complicating injuries, your doctor can reduce the pain by twisting the wrist so that the palm faces upward and then bending (flexing) the arm at the elbow. There is usually a click, and the child almost instantaneously begins to use the arm.

Knee sprains often occur during sporting events and may involve any one of a number of ligaments. These sprains may permit abnormally increased movement from side to side or from front to back. Or the knee may lock and not straighten. Sprains hurt immediately and usually continue to be painful, in contrast to the typical ligament tear, which is painful initially but resolves relatively rapidly.

Ankle sprains and fractures are very common, with the foot twisting either in or out. There is usually immediate pain and swelling. One place often hurts more than others when fractures are associated with sprains.

Caution

Since it is difficult to be certain that a bone is not fractured, it is usually wise to have the injury examined

Bone injuries may occur with other problems

Index

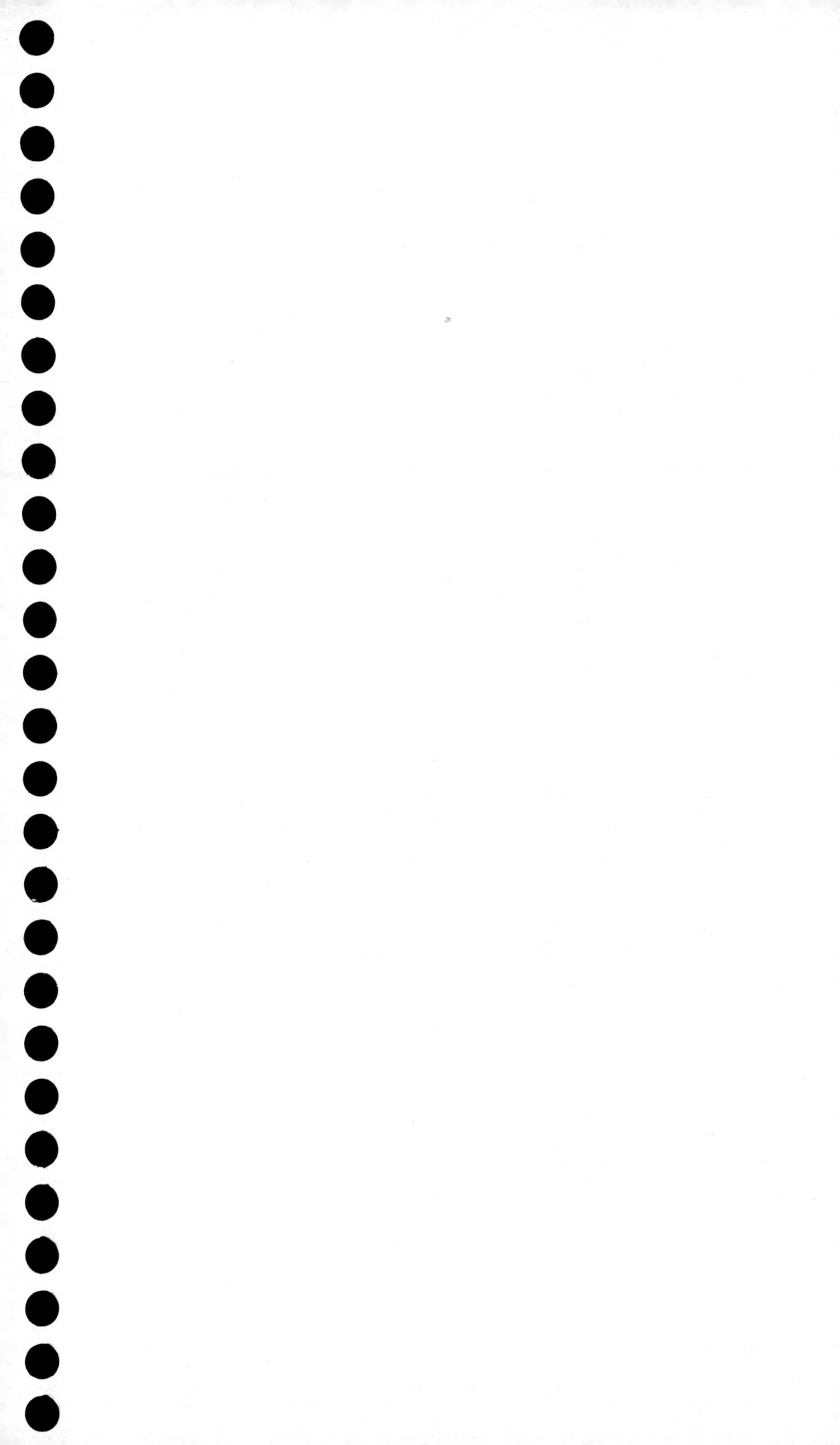

". . . probably the most comprehensive single medical textbook written on HIV disease."
—from a review of the first edition in Annals of Internal Medicine

THE AIDS KNOWLEDGE BASE:

A Textbook on HIV Disease from the University of California, San Francisco and the San Francisco General Hospital, Second Edition

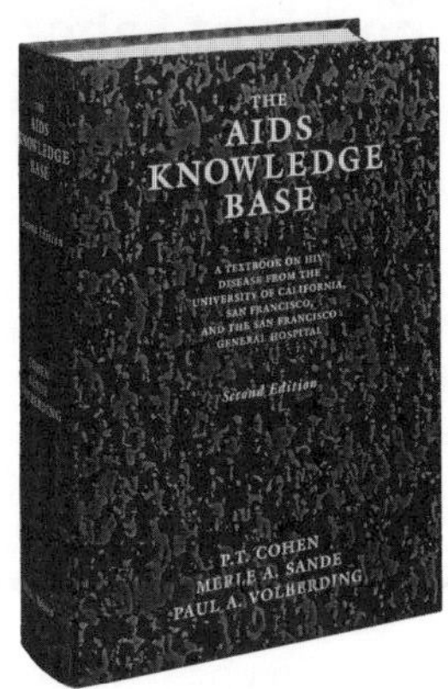

Edited by **P. T. Cohen, M.D., Ph.D.,** **Merle A. Sande, M.D.,** and **Paul A. Volberding, M.D.**

Published by the Massachusetts Medical Society in its first edition, the latest edition of this encyclopedic compendium is thoroughly revised and updated to give you:

- **Clinically tested and up-to-date strategies you can use to evaluate, manage, and treat HIV disease and associated problems**
- **A comprehensive guide to the current literature through extensive selected references**
- **A full, authoritative discussion of the ethical, legal, social, political, and fiscal implications of AIDS**

Authoritative. . .
This monumental work brings together 85 outstanding contributing authors who draw on more than a decade of unparalleled experience in treating HIV-related diseases at the University of California, San Francisco and the San Francisco General Hospital.

Complete. . .
From basic information to specific therapies, **THE AIDS KNOWLEDGE BASE, Second Edition,** is unsurpassed in its broad, current coverage of HIV disease. Extensive, current references at the end of each chapter point the way to detailed literature for deeper study of specific topics. **More than 200 charts, tables, and photos (including color) complete the text.**

THE AIDS KNOWLEDGE BASE, Second Edition, is an invaluable tool in combating HIV disease.

Scheduled for publication in Summer1994. Paperback, approx. 1,200 pages, illustrated, #770671, $125.00(T)

Available at your local medical bookstore or by calling toll-free 1(800)527-0145 (Mon. - Fri., 8:30-5:30 Eastern time) Call today for a Free 30–Day Trial!

LB
LITTLE, BROWN AND COMPANY
Medical Division
34 Beacon Street • Boston, MA 02108

M1362

Keep These Authoritative Guides by Your Side

Interpretation of Diagnostic Tests: A Synopsis of Laboratory Medicine, Fifth Edition

By **Jacques Wallach, M.D.**

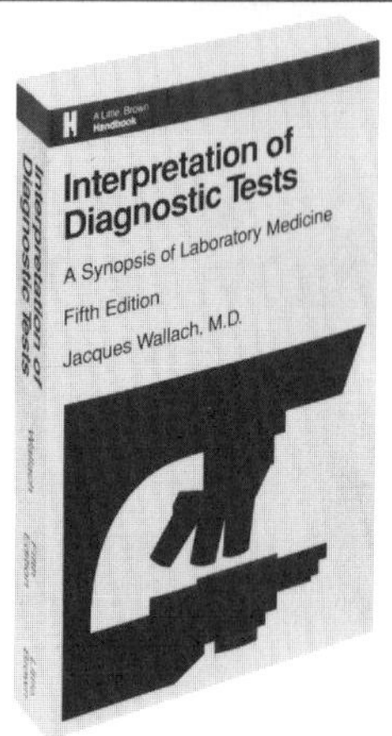

This popular handbook contains the most current information available on adult and pediatric laboratory tests. The book is conveniently divided into four sections, making it the ideal reference for on-the-spot consultation whenever you select or interpret laboratory tests.

The first section presents normal adult and pediatric values for common tests in both discussion and table formats. The second section covers specific lab exams with respect to the diseases or conditions in which test results are increased, normal, or decreased. Section Three lists 500 diseases by organ system, with abnormal and normal test findings. The final section shows you how test results may vary when a patient is taking a drug. For speedy consultation and current facts, **Interpretation of Diagnostic Tests, Fifth Edition,** is an indispensable companion.

1992. 960 pages, paperback, #920509, $36.50

HIV Infection: A Clinical Manual, Second Edition

Edited by **Howard Libman, M.D.**, and **Robert A. Witzburg, M.D.**

Written by internists for internists, this important manual is a practical guide to the full range of issues surrounding the diagnosis and treatment of the adult AIDS patient.

HIV Infection: A Clinical Manual offers a broad-based, multidisciplinary approach to the topic of HIV infected patients. Drs. Libman and Witzburg, in collaboration with 33 experts, present an overview of HIV infection, discuss epidemiology, explore clinical syndromes and clinical manifestations, and more. Numerous line drawings and photographs supplement the text, and useful tables and charts make information easily accessible.

1993. 576 pages, illustrated, paperback, #511625, $34.00

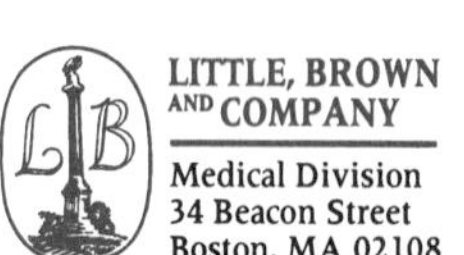

LITTLE, BROWN AND COMPANY
Medical Division
34 Beacon Street
Boston, MA 02108

Available at your local medical bookstore or by calling toll-free 1(800)527-0145 (Mon. - Fri., 8:30-5:30 Eastern time)